EXERCISE TESTING AND TRAINING
IN CORONARY HEART DISEASE

EXERCISE TESTING AND TRAINING
IN
CORONARY HEART DISEASE

JEAN-MARIE R. DETRY, M.D.

Agrégé de l'Enseignement Supérieur
Maître de Conférences à l'Université Catholique de Louvain

The Williams and Wilkins Company / Baltimore
H.E. Stenfert Kroese B.V. / Leiden
1973

Sole distributor for the United States of America and Canada
THE WILLIAMS AND WILKINS COMPANY / BALTIMORE

Copyright 1973
by H.E. Stenfert Kroese B.V., Publishers,
P.O. Box 33, Leiden, The Netherlands.
ISBN-13: 978-90-207-0374-0   e-ISBN-13: 978-94-010-2361-0
DOI: 10.1007/978-94-010-2361-0

To Francette
Pierre
Marc

Author's address :
Cardiopulmonary Laboratory,
University Hospital,
Brusselsestraat, 69,
3000 Louvain (Belgium)

FOREWORD

*This study on « Exercise testing and training in coronary heart disease »
is a remarkable compilation of numerous research studies, primarily from laboratories in Europe and the United States over the last decade or more. The
topic reflects a growing awareness of and concern about the rapidly expanding
understanding of the pathophysiology of coronary atherosclerotic heart disease.
Since muscular exercise increases aerobic metabolism of myocardial and working
skeletal muscles, greater flow of oxygenated blood is required by each; yet
underlying vascular disease restricts these responses. This implicit paradox
is here considered forthrightly. Examination of these relationships in symptomatic
patients requires care and caution, because of the potential and occasionally
real risks entailed. Accordingly, indirect assessment, particularly by noninvasive
techniques, becomes increasingly important to detecting and monitoring - for
the safety of the patients studied - the evidence of myocardial ischemia and
impairment of left ventricular function under stress. Adequate assessment requires
well-designed experimental studies to quantify true relationships and to measure
the limits of functional capacity and the mechanisms of its impairment. Furthermore, alterations can be induced by therapy, whether this be pharmacological,
medical or surgical, or achieved by physical reconditioning through exercise
training.*

*Not only is the cardiovascular system impaired by discrete and diffuse vascular
lesions at central sites, but the degree of impairment is dynamic rather than
static. It is dynamic because of progressive changes in the severity of coronary
atherosclerosis, in clinical manifestations of myocardial dysfunction and in
the sum of whatever integrated hemodynamic loads are applied. Acute drug
therapy, (i.e., nitroglycerin) and the chronic effects of compensatory adaptive
mechanisms modify these changes. The final integration of all interacting factors
is most reliably measured in a functional sense by maximal oxygen intake.
However, documentation that such measurements are indeed maximal, especially
when they can be altered acutely and reversibly - in coronary patients - by
pharmacologically induced changes in ventricular loading, requires careful
design of experimental methods and a broad understanding of physiological
regulatory and control mechanisms. Thus, there is a dilemma in terminology;
are the observed peak values of oxygen intake under conditions of « symptom-
limited » voluntary performance indeed « maximal » or are they not?*

*There appear to be at least two other dynamic aspects of the pathophysiology,
or trends in longitudinal manifestations of pathophysiology with natural history
of disease. One of these is the changing predictive power and diagnostic significance of the ST depression in response to exercise. As disease progresses,
and particularly after massive or recurrent myocardial infarction with survival,
there is significant impairment of contractile power and synergy of the left*

ventricle. Dr. Detry has extensively reviewed the evidence and indicated the need for further investigation of the possible role of akinesis and dyskinesis as well as asynergy in contributing to these changes expressed in early repolarization forces of the ECG. The other is the divergent adaptation to physical training in middle-age. In health, stroke volume increases, but in patients with coronary disease investigators report changes primarily in $a-\bar{v}_{O_2}$ difference or in stroke volume: the importance of evolving changes in adaptation after infarction alluted to by Dr. Detry offers, for the first time, a plausible explanation.

Given these considerations, the organization and careful preparation of this book reveals an extensive knowledge of the relevant literature. Of greater importance are the new data contributed by Dr. Detry. Both are presented with a perspective that can only be achieved after most intensive personal review, analysis and participation in many facets of experimental research and clinical investigation of the highest quality. The reader is easily guided through a massive amount of investigative efforts by a wellconceived outline of important items. Yet at all times the identity and chronology of the sources, and the substantive data are documented. In areas where general consensus and understanding have not yet emerged, Dr. Detry indicates his awareness of the uncertainties. In a word, this is the work of a well trained investigator. For patients involved with disease, it will aid the understanding of the physicians who manage their problems.

It is particularly gratifying to the undersigned to have had the opportunity and pleasure of joining with others in the rigorous preparation of Dr. Jean-Marie R. Detry for an academic career of excellence. Given the magnificient redaction of this study as evidence, I look forward with high expectations that he will continue to add important insights and understanding to the pathophysiology of coronary disease in the future.

ROBERT A. BRUCE, M.D.
Professor of Medicine
Director, Division of Cardiology
University of Washington, Seattle.

CONTENTS

INTRODUCTION

Coronary heart disease represents a major medical problem since it is the most important cause of morbidity and mortality in the middle-aged and old population ; recent statistics also indicate an increasing incidence of coronary heart disease which is tending to become more frequent in younger age groups. Sustained efforts by epidemiologists in the recent years have helped to define the etiologic factors, to identify the most common risk factors and to propose some preventive measures which hopefully will limit the extension of this disease ; extensive clinical research has also led to substantial improvements in the medical and surgical treatment of acute and chronic coronary insufficiency.

The first step in the management of a coronary patient is a correct diagnosis ; the medical history, the clinical examination and the resting electrocardiogram do not always provide sufficient objective data to reach the right diagnosis and exercise testing has become a common and most useful extension of the clinical examination of a patient in whom coronary heart disease is suspected. Besides electrocardiographic data, exercise testing also provides most precious information about the patient's functional capacity which cannot be adequately estimated from resting measurements. Since abnormal exertional electrocardiogram in apparently healthy subjects is attended by a subsequent high incidence of clinical coronary heart disease, exercise electrocardiography is now used to detect latent coronary heart disease with the hope of preventing its evolution to clinical disease.

Since many years the medical treatment of stabilized coronary heart disease includes the nitrate compounds, the anticoagulants and the sedatives; introduction of beta-blocking agents was a genuine major therapeutical advance and extensive research is now devoted to new pharmacological compounds which may increase the myocardial blood flow and/or improve the myocardial metabolism. The importance of hygieno-dietetic prescriptions designed to influence risk factors such as overweight, abnormal blood lipids level, high blood pressure and smoking, is also increasingly clear. The valuable effects of physical activity and training in healthy subjects have logically led to study the effects of physical training in coronary patients. These studies have revealed that supervised physical activity was beneficial to many patients with overt clinical coronary disease and indicated that the former attitude of suspicion about physical activity in coronary patients was often not justified ; supervised physical training has accordingly become an important aspect of the management of coronary patients.

The present study reviews some important aspects of exercise testing and training in coronary heart disease and the emphasis has deliberately been placed on those aspects which are the most familiar to the author. Three aspects of the adaptation to exercise will be given particular consideration, namely the electrocardiographic response to submaximal and maximal exercise, the hemodynamic adjustments during submaximal exercise, and the maximal exercise capacity, better designated as physical work capacity. The adaptation to exercise of coronary patients can be modified by several therapeutics and a special attention will be given to the effects of nitroglycerin and to those of physical training.

To clarify the presentation, the pathophysiological basis, methods and results of exercise electrocardiography (Chapter 2) have been reviewed separately from those of the determination of the physical work capacity (Chapter 3) while a separate chapter is devoted to physical training. This separation into chapters is largely artificial since many points are in fact common to these topics. In order to facilitate understanding, some basic physiological principles have been reviewed in the first chapter while reference to specific data collected in normal subjects is made further on when necessary. Most of the author's original data have been previously published and they will not be further detailed here. The bibliography has deliberately been limited to papers or books published in the recent years and to some earlier classical contributions.

CHAPTER I

Physiological considerations

Physiological response to exercise is complex and based on many adjustments involving different organs and systems, as the muscles, the nervous system and the cardiorespiratory system. From a cardiovascular point of view, the purpose of these adjustments is to supply more oxygen and fuel to the working muscles and to eliminate the waste products resulting from the increased metabolic activity. In this respect, the role of the respiratory system is essential: the pulmonary function does not however limit the exercise capacity of normal subjects at sea level, and it will not be discussed here. Under normal conditions the cardiac response to exercise is probably not limited by myocardial hypoxia : the latter does however become a major limiting factor in patients with coronary heart disease.

This introductory chapter deals firstly with the cardiovascular response to exercise and the factors which may affect this response, and secondly with the regulation of the coronary blood flow and the determinants of myocardial oxygen consumption.

CARDIOVASCULAR RESPONSE TO EXERCISE

According to the Fick principle, the oxygen consumption ($\dot{V}_{O2}$) is equal to the product of the cardiac output (heart rate x stroke volume) and the total arterial-mixed venous oxygen difference ($a\text{-}\bar{v}_{O2}$) :

$$\dot{V}_{O2} = \text{heart rate x stroke volume x } a\text{-}\bar{v}_{O2} \text{ difference}$$
$$\text{beats/min} \qquad \text{ml/beat} \qquad \text{ml/l}$$

Increased oxygen consumption during exercise will consequently be based on two mechanisms : (1) an increase in the cardiac output ; depending on the conditions, the increase in cardiac output will result from increments in stroke volume and/or in heart rate ; (2) a widening of the total $a\text{-}\bar{v}_{O2}$ difference due to a greater extraction of the oxygen from the blood by the working muscles ; the redistribution of cardiac output with exercise, which makes more blood available for the active muscles, also plays an important role in the increase of the total $a\text{-}\bar{v}_{O2}$ difference. These adaptive mechanisms are closely connected with the regulation of the systemic blood pressure, which also depends on the cardiac output response and on changes in its distribution.

The cardio-vascular response to exercise is influenced by several factors, in particular the type of exercise (leg or arm exercise ; dynamic or isometric work), the age of the subject, the duration of the exercise and the environmental conditions. In the daily life, the most common type of exercise is dynamic exercise performed with the legs, and this type of work has been studied most extensively ; exercise testing and training are also based on such exercise. The cardiovascular response to dynamic leg exercise is consequently reviewed first and the physiological mechanisms involved in this response are discussed. Subsequently, several of the factors affecting the cardio-vascular response to exercise are briefly considered.

A. Dynamic leg exercise.

1. Increased transport of oxygen.

Increased transport of oxygen during exercise results mostly from an increased cardiac output. The contributions of the heart rate and the stroke volume to the increments in cardiac output vary according to the posture and the intensity of the exercise (Bevegard et al., 1960, 1963 ; Chapman et al., 1960 ; Wang et al., 1960 ; Holmgren et al., 1960).

In the resting supine posture, the cardiac output is approximately 2 liters/min higher than in the resting upright posture, due to greater stroke volume values (Bevegard et al., 1960). During submaximal

6

exercise in supine position, the stroke volume does not change, or increases only slightly (Bevegard et al., 1960, 1963 ; Holmgren et al., 1960), and the increase in cardiac output depends essentially on the increase in heart rate (fig. 1). During supine exercise,

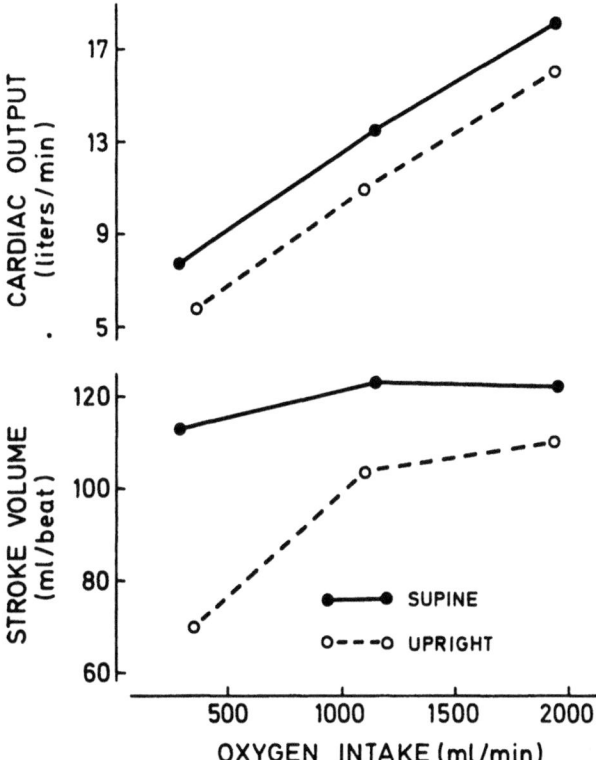

Fig. 1. — Cardiac output and stroke volume at rest and during exercise in supine and upright postures in 7 normal young males (drawn from data of Holmgren et al., 1960).

the heart rate and the cardiac output increase therefore linearly with the oxygen consumption (Holmgren et al., 1960) ; it is however not known whether or not this relationship remains linear up to maximal exercise levels (Marshall and Shepherd, 1968).

At the onset of upright exercise, both the heart rate and the stroke volume contribute to the increase in cardiac output (Bevegard et al., 1960, 1963). At a given level of submaximal oxygen consumption, however, the cardiac output remains lower than in supine posture (fig. 1) ; this postural difference tends to be less marked at high levels of exercise (Bevegard et al., 1963). During upright exercise, the maximal values of stroke volume are usually reached at an exercise intensity corresponding to 40 - 50 % of the maximal oxygen intake (Åstrand et al., 1965 ; Grimby

et al., 1966 ; Ekblom and Hermansen, 1968 ; Hartley et al., 1969) but there are exceptions to this general rule (Ekblom et al., 1968 ; Saltin et al., 1968 ; Hermansen et al., 1970). The maximal values of upright stroke volume often exceed those of the resting supine stroke volume and this difference can reach 20 to 23 % (Grimby et al., 1966 ; Hartley et al., 1969). During upright exercise, the heart rate and the cardiac output are linearly related to the oxygen consumption up to approximately 70 % of the maximal oxygen intake ; at higher exercise levels, the contribution of the increase of $a\text{-}\bar{v}_{O_2}$ difference appears greater than that of the increase in cardiac output (Åstrand et al., 1964 ; Bevegard and Shepherd, 1967).

Exercise is attended by hemoconcentration proportionate to the intensity of the exercise (Bevegard et al., 1960 ; Ekblom et al., 1968 ; Hartley et al., 1969), which leads to higher arterial oxygen capacity. This also contributes to the increased transport of oxygen since the arterial oxygen saturation remains within normal limits during exercise in sedentary subjects (Mitchell et al., 1958 ; Rowell et al., 1964b) ; a decrease of the arterial oxygen saturation at maximal exercise has, however, been observed in athletes (Rowell et al., 1964b).

2. Widening of the total $a\text{-}\bar{v}_{O_2}$ difference.

The total $a\text{-}\bar{v}_{O_2}$ difference results from the mixing in the cardiac cavities of blood coming from parts of the body which have different local $a\text{-}\bar{v}_{O_2}$ differences. It consequently depends on the distribution of the cardiac output among the various regions and on their respective metabolic activity. The total $a\text{-}\bar{v}_{O_2}$ difference increases with the severity of the exercise ; in upright posture the $a\text{-}\bar{v}_{O_2}$ difference is linearly related to the relative intensity of the exercise (Åstrand et al., 1964). In supine posture, the relationship between submaximal oxygen consumption and total $a\text{-}\bar{v}_{O_2}$ difference appears to be hyperbolic (Denolin et al., 1966 ; Bevegard and Shepherd, 1967).

The evolution during leg exercise of the femoral $a\text{-}\bar{v}_{O_2}$ difference is not clear. Reeves et al. (1961a) have indeed reported that in the resting upright posture, the femoral $a\text{-}\bar{v}_{O_2}$ difference was already nearly maximal and that the increased oxygen consumption of the muscles was mostly dependent on an increase in the femoral flow. Others have however demonstrated the increase in the total $a\text{-}\bar{v}_{O_2}$ difference during upright exercise to be paralleled by an increase in the femoral $a\text{-}\bar{v}_{O_2}$ difference, which would reflect a progressively greater extraction of the oxygen from the blood by the working muscles (Rowell, 1962 ;

Saltin et al., 1968); this adaptive mechanism seems to be effective also in supine posture (Reeves et al., 1961b). The widening of the $a\text{-}\bar{v}_{O_2}$ difference is facilitated by a shift to the right of the oxygen dissociation curve which is due to the lower p_H, higher p_{CO_2} and higher temperature.

3. Redistribution of the cardiac output.

The distribution of cardiac output is drastically modified by exercise (table 1). The muscle blood flow represents only 20 % of the resting cardiac output but during exercise muscle blood flow becomes a progressively greater part of the cardiac output, finally representing approximately 90 % of the total cardiac output during maximal exercise (Wade and Bishop, 1962). This increase in the muscle blood flow results from the increase in the cardiac output and also from its redistribution away from non active regions, i.e. the splanchnic organs and kidneys (Wade and Bishop, 1962 ; Bevegard and Shepherd, 1967 ; Rowell, 1971). At rest the splanchnic and renal flows represent 40-45 % of the total cardiac output and the $a\text{-}\bar{v}_{O_2}$ difference across these vascular beds is small. During exercise the splanchnic and renal flows decrease (Rowell et al., 1964a ; Grimby, 1965 ; Castenfors and Piscator, 1967) and the $a\text{-}\bar{v}_{O_2}$ difference across these regions increase accordingly : this adaptive mecanism is important since it contributes significantly to the increase in muscle blood flow and so to the increase in the total $a\text{-}\bar{v}_{O_2}$ difference. For instance, a reduction of the splanchnic and renal flows from 2.5 liters/min at rest to 0.5 liters/min at the maximal exercise level makes 2 liters/min of oxygenated blood available for the working muscles and this, assuming a peripheral oxygen extraction of 80 % and an arterial oxygen content of 21 ml/100 ml, correspond to approximately 350 ml of oxygen.

These adjustments of splanchnic and renal flows during exercise are linearly related to the percentage of the maximal oxygen consumption required (relative work load) and not to the absolute oxygen intake (Rowell et al., 1964a ; Grimby, 1965). For an athlete, who has a very high maximal oxygen intake, a given level of oxygen consumption represents a smaller relative work load than for a sedentary person ; at the same absolute workload, however, athletes and sedentary subjects have the same cardiac output (Bevegard et al., 1963). Thus at any absolute level of oxygen intake the athlete will have higher splanchnic and renal flows than the sedentary subject ; since they have similar cardiac output, the fraction of this cardiac output available for the muscles must be lower in the athletes. At a given level of oxygen intake, the muscle blood flow (per 100 g of muscle) appears indeed to be lower in well trained subjects compared to sedentary persons (Grimby et al., 1967), which supports the view that athletes have a lower total muscle blood flow, if we assume that for the same absolute exercise their active muscle mass is similar. At the same level of relative energy expenditure, however, athletes and sedentary persons seem to have the same muscle blood flow per 100 g (Grimby et al., 1967).

During exercise, the cerebral blood flow remains constant (Wade and Bishop, 1962). The skin blood

TABLE 1

Distribution of cardiac output at rest and during maximal exercise in normal subjects (from Wade and Bishop, 1962).

	Rest		Maximal exercise	
	Blood flow ml/min	% of cardiac output	Blood flow ml/min	% of cardiac output
Splanchnic	1400	24 %	300	1 %
Renal	1100	19 %	250	1 %
Cerebral	750	13 %	750	3 %
Coronary	250	4 %	1000	4 %
Skeletal Muscle	1200	21 %	22000	88 %
Skin	500	9 %	600	2.5 %
Other organs	600	10 %	100	0.4 %
Cardiac output	5800		25000	

flow depends on the intensity of the exercise. During submaximal exercise, the flow to the skin is increased to facilitate the dissipation of heat (Wade and Bishop, 1962 ; Bevegard and Shepherd, 1966a) ; the total flow to the resting forearm is not increased however, which indicates a redistribution of blood flow from the inactive muscles to the skin during exercise (Bevegard and Shepherd, 1966a). But during strenuous or maximal exercise, which is marked by extreme pallor of the skin, the skin blood flow decreases while the flow to the inactive muscles is further reduced (Bevegard and Shepherd, 1966a ; Saltin et al., 1968) ; these adjustments contribute to increase the portion of the maximal cardiac output directed to the active muscles. These adaptations of the skin circulation in fact represent a balance between the requirements of the thermoregulation and the need to increase the muscle blood flow as much as possible. The regulation of the coronary blood flow during exercise will be discussed later in this chapter.

4. Adaptative mechanisms.

The mechanisms involved in the cardiovascular adaptation to exercise are complex and not yet fully understood (Bevegard and Shepherd, 1967 ; Braunwald et al., 1967 ; Guyton, 1967 ; Shepherd, 1967). As soon as exercise is started, the blood vessels in the working muscles dilate ; this decrease of the skeletal muscle vascular resistance, which is proportional to the metabolic activity, is likely to be under local control. The agents responsible for the local regulation of blood flow through the muscles during exercise are still being discussed. The muscle blood flow is probably not regulated by a single factor but rather by a combination of factors among which the roles of hypoxia and potassium appear essential (Skinner and Powell, 1967 ; Haddy and Scott, 1968) ; other agents such as adenosine nucleotides may also play a role (Haddy and Scott, 1968). This sudden decrease in resistance to flow through the active muscles requires rapidly adaptive changes to prevent a fall in the systemic pressure : these adjustments are an immediate rise in cardiac output and a change in its distribution.

Venous return to the right side of the heart is increased immediately by the action of the muscle pump and abdomino-thoracic pump ; these mechanisms are combined with a generalized constriction of the capacity vessels (Bevegard and Shepherd, 1965, 1966a). This increase in the tension of the venous walls in both exercising and non exercising limbs is mediated by sympathetic noradrenergic nerves and is proportional to the severity of the exercise. The increase in venous tone with exercise reduces the amount of blood contained in the capacity vessels and contributes to increase the venous return (Bevegard and Shepherd, 1967 ; Shepherd, 1967).

The cardiac output response to exercise is based on the interaction of several mechanisms, notably the tachycardia, the sympathetic stimulation and the Frank-Starling mechanism (Braunwald et al., 1967a). The increase in stroke volume or the persistance of an unchanged stroke volume at a faster heart rate is achieved partly through increased myocardial contractility ; the latter is related to increased sympathetic stimulation of the heart and to the higher heart rate itself. The Frank-Starling mechanism also plays a role in the evolution of stroke volume during exercise : for a given value of heart rate, the stroke volume and the end-diastolic volume of the heart are indeed greater during mild supine exercise than during resting tachycardia induced by atrial pacing (Braunwald et al., 1967a). During supine exercise the role of the Frank-Starling mechanism is masked by the faster heart rate so that the heart volume does not increase or decreases slightly (Holmgren and Ovenfors, 1960 ; Braunwald et al., 1967a) ; unfortunately, no data on heart volume are available during upright exercise, where the contribution of the Frank-Starling mechanism must be greater than during supine exercise (Holmgren and Ovenfors, 1960 ; Braunwald et al., 1967a). In the absence of one of the above mentioned mechanisms, cardiac output can still rise during submaximal exercise but all three adaptive mechanisms are required for a normal cardiac output response to maximal exercise (Epstein et al., 1965 ; Braunwald et al., 1967a).

Despite the fall in total peripheral resistance which occurs during exercise, the mean arterial pressure increases moderately, and this increase in arterial pressure is related to the severity of the exercise (Åstrand et al., 1965). Maintenance of systemic pressure during exercise depends on the increase in cardiac output and on the vasoconstriction of the resistance vessels in the non-exercising beds (Bevegard and Shepherd, 1967 ; Shepherd, 1967). This reflex vasoconstriction, presumably mediated by increased sympathetic tone (Bevegard et al., 1966a), also contributes to the redistribution of the cardiac output by causing a decrease of the flow to the non active beds (Rowell et al., 1964 ; Grimby, 1965 ; Bevegard et al., 1966a) ; in the working muscles, the increased sympathetic activity is overcome by local potent vasodilating factors, with as a net result an increase in the flow. Increased tone of the resistance vessels in the non-working limbs probably explains why exercise performed with small muscle groups (arm exercise, for instance), is attended by a greater increase in mean blood pressure (Åstrand et al., 1965 ; Bevegard et al., 1966a ; Bevegard and Shepherd, 1967 ; Shepherd, 1967 ; Stenberg et al., 1967) ; the dilated vascular bed is smaller in this type of work.

Higher blood pressure during exercise represents a stimulus for the baroreceptor ; the baroreceptors continue to oppose the rise in heart rate and blood pressure but the carotid sinus mechanism is over-ridden by exercise stimuli (Bevegard et al., 1966b).

The cardiovascular response to exercise is thus the result of coordinated changes involving the heart, the resistance vessels and the capacity vessels ; these changes are mediated by local mechanisms causing the fall in vascular resistance in the working muscles, by the fundamental characteristics of the heart and by an increased activity of the sympathetic system. The latter is responsible for the increased tone of the capacitance vessels and of the resistance vessels in the non active beds, and partly explains the higher heart rate and the increased myocardial contractility; the receptors and afferent pathways concerned with the reflex increased activity of the sympathetic system are however still unknown (Bevegard and Shepherd, 1967).

B. Isometric exercise.

Isometric exercise or static effort may be defined as a sustained muscular contraction against a fixed resistance, and is involved in many common activities such as lifting, holding or pushing objects. The cardiovascular response to this type of exercise is characterized by higher increments in heart rate, cardiac output and blood pressure as compared to dynamic exercise of the same absolute intensity (Lind et al., 1966 ; Lind, 1970) ; also, in normal subjects, the left ventricular end-diastolic pressure does not change or rises only slightly while the stroke work increases significantly (Mullins et al., 1970 ; Helfant et al., 1971b ; Kivowitz et al., 1971). The increase in blood pressure is proportionate to the intensity of the sustained contraction (fraction of the maximal voluntary contraction) and its duration, but not to the mass of skeletal muscle involved : a similar degree of static effort will therefore produce the same pressure load whether performed by small forearm muscles or by much larger leg muscles (Lind et al., 1966).

The rise in pressure during isometric exercise is related to the increments in heart rate and cardiac output since total systemic resistance does not change or decreases only slightly. The blood pressure response to isometric exercise appears to be under control of a reflex which originates in the muscle itself, perhaps under the influence of released potassium (Lind et al., 1966) ; this reflex is powerful since combination of static exercise and dynamic work causes additive responses of blood pressure, heart rate and probably cardiac output (Lind et al., 1966 ; Lind, 1970). Sustained isometric handgrip exercise is now used as a stress test for evaluation of the left ventricular function since the hemodynamic response of patients with heart disease is significantly different from that of normal subjects (Mullins et al., 1970 ; Helfant et al., 1971b ; Kivowitz et al., 1971).

At a given level of oxygen intake, rhythmic exercise performed with the arms is also attended by higher heart rate and blood pressure than dynamic leg exercise, while cardiac output is the same ; the more important static work involved in arm exercise probably contributes to this difference (Åstrand et al., 1965 ; Stenberg et al., 1967).

C. Prolonged and repeated exercise.

During prolonged exercise at a constant workload, the cardiovascular adjustments described above are progressively modified. As exercise is prolonged over 10 minutes, there is a gradual decrease in stroke volume with a compensatory increase in heart rate to keep the cardiac output almost constant ; simultaneously, the right ventricular end-diastolic pressure, the mean pulmonary arterial pressure and the systemic arterial pressure fall (Cobb and Johnson, 1963 ; Saltin and Stenberg, 1964 ; Ekelund, 1967b ; Sowton and Burkart, 1967). These hemodynamic changes occur during prolonged moderate or heavy exercise, both in supine and upright position (Ekelund and Holmgren, 1964 ; Ekelund, 1966 ; Ekelund, 1967a). The mechanisms responsible for these adjustments are still the subject of discussion.

The major change appears to be a progressive decline in the tone the capacitance vessels causing a shift of blood away from the central vasculature ; this gradual increase in the compliance of the veins is probably responsible for the decrease in cardiac filling pressure and stroke volume, while the cardiac output is maintained by an increase in heart rate (Ekelund, 1967b; Rowell, 1972). The decline in systemic pressure and resistance might result from a dilatation of the resistance vessels of the skin (Saltin and Stenberg, 1964). All these adjustments combine to redistribute part of the circulating blood volume to superficial regions, facilitating heat loss, and they may result from the increasing thermoregulatory needs during prolonged exercise; the increase in heart rate during prolonged exercise is indeed attended by an increase in oesophageal temperature, and both these changes are abolished when exercise is performed at low ambiant temperature (Kitzing et al., 1968). An alternative explanation for the decrease in stroke volume during prolonged exercise is a progressive alteration of the myocardial function (Saltin and Stenberg, 1964).

The hemodynamic drift with prolonged exercise is very similar to that occuring when a given submaximal exercise is repeated after a short rest interval (Burkart et al., 1967), when prolonged intermittent work is performed (Detry et al., 1972a) or when light work is performed after heavy exertion (Hartley and Saltin, 1968). As for prolonged exercise, the mechanisms involved in these hemodynamic modifications are not yet fully understood; the changes in heart rate during repeated exercise are related to changes in oesophageal temperature, but the evidence for a causal relationship is still lacking (Detry et al., 1972a). Hartley et al. (1970) have recently proposed that the withdrawal of the parasympathetic tone may play a role in the highest heart rate noted during submaximal exercise preceded by heavy exertion.

Higher heart rate and lower stroke volume and blood pressure with repetition of submaximal exercise have to be kept in mind in the design of experimental protocols. When maximal exercise is repeated after half an hour's rest, the maximal heart rate is not significantly modified, however (Detry and Bruce, 1971a).

D. Environmental factors.

Exercise performed in the heat is characterized by a higher heart rate and lower stroke volume, central blood volume and blood pressure (Brouha et al., 1960 ; Williams et al., 1962 ; Rowell et al., 1966); the cardiac output is either unchanged or increased (Rowell et al., 1969) when body heating is direct and intense. These hemodynamic modifications probably result from a decreased tone of the capacitance vessels with peripheral displacement of circulating blood volume ; this is supported by the abolition of the venomotor response when exercise is performed in the heat (Bevegard and Shepherd, 1965 ; Rowell et al., 1971a ; 1971b). Circulatory modifications due to heat stress are less marked in physically well trained subjects and are reduced after heat acclimatization (Robinson S., 1967 ; Rowell et al., 1967 ; Brouwers et al., 1968).

Exposure to a low environmental temperature, at rest or during exercise, does not modify heart rate or cardiac output but causes a rise in systemic pressure (Epstein et al., 1969 ; Leon et al., 1970). Increased total peripheral resistance in a cold environment appears to be related to a thermoregulatory response causing cutaneous vasoconstriction ; changes in total conductance in the cold indicate however that other organs than the skin must be involved in this response.

E. Influence of sex and age.

The most important difference between the sexes is that during exercise of the same absolute intensity, women have a lower stroke volume and a higher heart rate compared with men. The lower stroke volume of women during exercise is related to their lower heart volume (Åstrand et al., 1964). Åstrand et al. (1964) suggested that, at a given oxygen intake, women had a higher cardiac output than men, but this sex difference has not been confirmed by later studies (Saltin et al., 1968 ; Hartley et al., 1969 ; Kiblom and Åstrand, 1971); for the same absolute level of submaximal exercise, women consequently have the same total $a\text{-}\bar{v}_{O_2}$ difference as men but, due to their lower oxygen capacity, the O_2 saturation of their mixed pulmonary venous blood is lower.

Aging progressively alters the cardiovascular response to exercise. At a given level of submaximal oxygen intake, old subjects of both sexes have a lower cardiac output and a greater $a\text{-}\bar{v}_{O_2}$ difference than younger subjects ; this difference, already present at rest, results from the decrease of the stroke volume with age (Strandell, 1964 ; Julius et al., 1967 ; Kiblom and Åstrand, 1971). Resting arterial blood pressure and systemic resistance are higher in old age and they increase to a greater extent during exercise than in younger subjects (Strandell, 1964 ; Julius et al., 1967 ; Kiblom and Åstrand, 1971); this probably reflects decreased elasticity of arterial wall with aging (Marshall and Shepherd, 1968).

CORONARY BLOOD FLOW AND THE DETERMINANTS OF MYOCARDIAL OXYGEN CONSUMPTION

At rest, the myocardium extracts 75 % of the oxygen supplied by the coronary blood flow (Messer et al., 1962). The resting intramyocardial partial pressure in O_2 (P_{O_2}) as reflected by the P_{O_2} of the coronary sinus blood, is low and averages 20 mm Hg : the intramyocardial P_{O_2} is not uniform, however, and it is probably as low as 10 mm Hg in the subendocardial regions (Moss, 1968). In these conditions, increase in myocardial oxygen consumption (MV_{O_2}) will depend essentially on increase in coronary blood flow rather than on greater myocardial oxygen extraction.

Since the metabolism of the normal heart is based almost exclusively on aerobic processes (Scheuer, 1967; Neill, 1968 ; Nasser, 1970), very precise regulatory mechanisms are required for constant adjustment of the oxygen supply to the myocardium, i.e. the coronary blood flow, to the myocardial oxygen requirements. The mechanisms involved in the regulation of the coronary blood flow are described below and the factors which determine the myocardial oxygen consumption (MV_{O_2}) will be considered subsequently.

A. The regulation of the coronary blood flow.

Coronary blood flow is determined by the ratio of the effective perfusion pressure and the coronary vascular resistance. The factors regulating coronary blood flow can schematically be classified as physical, neural, neurohumoral and metabolic. All recent reviews agree in assigning the primary role to local. metabolic factors (Berne, 1964 ; Haddy and Scott, 1968 ; Gorlin, 1971 ; Lammerant, 1972).

1. Metabolic factors.

Myocardial blood flow is very sensitive to hypoxia ; increased oxygen consumption of the myocardium or decreased supply of oxygen to the myocardium is indeed promptly followed by an increase in coronary blood flow due to a fall in the coronary vascular resistance. These changes in coronary vascular resistance which maintain a constant balance between myocardial oxygen consumption and supply of oxygen to the myocardium appear to be under local metabolic control. The intramyocardial P_{O_2} is probably the most important factor regulating the coronary blood flow through the release of vasodilating metabolites (Berne, 1964 ; Haddy and Scott, 1968 ; Gorlin, 1971).

Berne and his group have proposed adenosine as the mediating substance and suggested (Berne, 1964 ; Rubio and Berne, 1969) the following scheme for metabolic regulation of coronary blood flow (fig. 2).

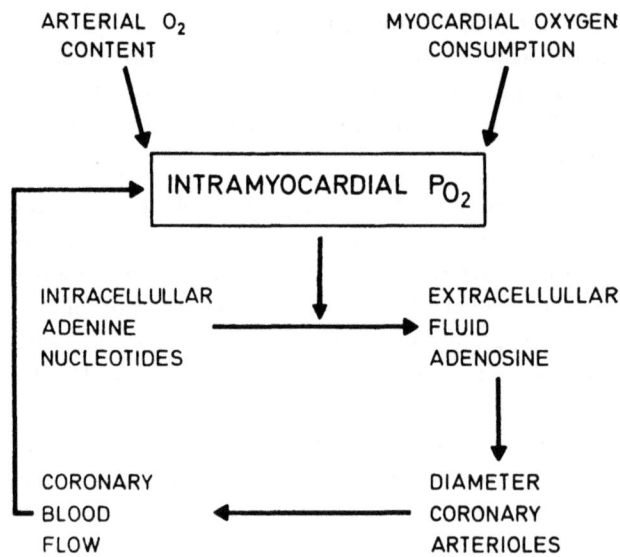

Fig. 2. — Berne's hypothesis on metabolic regulation of coronary blood flow (Berne, 1964).

Myocardial hypoxia disturbs the balance between synthesis and breakdown of ATP which leads to the accumulation of adenylic acid (AMP) and inorganic phosphate in the myocardial cell. Part of the AMP so formed is dephosphorylated to adenosine by the action of 5' nucleotidase in the cell membrane and reaches the interstitial fluid where it dilates the resistance vessels. The resulting increased coronary blood flow restores the intramyocardial P_{O_2}, decreases the formation of AMP, and washes out the adenosine from the interstitial fluid ; adenosine either re-enters the myocardial cell membrane to be transformed into AMP and inosine or is inactivated to inosine in the red cells. This mechanism is effective not only in hypoxic myocardium but under normal conditions as well : adenosine is indeed continuously released in the myocardial interstitial fluid and the concentration of adenosine appears to be the factor adjusting the coronary blood flow to the oxygen needs of the heart (Rubio and Berne, 1969).

The intramyocardial P_{O_2} decreases from the epicardium to the endocardium (Moss, 1968). The lower subendocardial P_{O_2} appears to result on one hand from the greater myocardial oxygen consumption due to the greater tension developed in the deep part of the ventricle, and on the other hand from the possibly lower subendocardial flow secondary to the higher subendocardial extravascular resistance. This gradient in P_{O_2} across the left ventricular wall might explain the frequent subendocardial location of myocardial ischemia (Gorlin, 1971 ; Lammerant, 1972).

Whether or not adenosine is the true and only metabolite regulating coronary blood flow has still to be established ; other factors such as potassium, hydrogen or oxygen per se are also perhaps involved (Haddy and Scott, 1968 ; Gorlin, 1971). In any event there is now convincing evidence for a potent local feedback mechanism assuring a constant balance between myocardial oxygen needs and supply.

2. Physical factors.

Coronary blood flow is determined by the coronary perfusion pressure and the intramyocardial pressure, also termed extravascular compression or resistance. Maintenance of aortic pressure is essential to increase coronary blood flow when the coronary vascular resistance is decreased ; during exercise, increase in aortic blood pressure certainly contributes to increase the coronary blood flow. A sudden increase in coronary perfusion pressure causes a transient increase in coronary blood flow, but due to autoregulation, the flow rapidly returns to control values despite sustained high perfusion pressure (Berne, 1964). Although of great importance in the determination of the coronary blood flow, the perfusion pressure does not appear to be an important factor in the regulation of coronary blood flow (Berne, 1964 ; Gorlin, 1971).

During cardiac cycle, variations in intramyocardial pressure cause phasic variations in the coronary blood flow (fig. 3). During isovolumetric contraction, the left coronary inflow is suddenly reduced and the flow can even be reversed ; during systole the left coronary inflow follows approximately the aortic pressure until early diastole where it suddenly increases. The duration of the diastole and the level of diastolic pressure are therefore important determinants of the left coronary flow. The right coronary flow follows a similar pattern, but due to the lower pressure developed in systole by the right ventricle, the flow is never abolished and the greater proportion of the right coronary blood flow occurs therefore during systole. The squeezing action of the ventricular contraction expels the blood from the capillaries and the small veins so that the coronary sinus blood flow is maximal during systole (Berne and Levy, 1967).

Direct measurements of intramyocardial pressure have demonstrated that it is higher in the deep subendocardial part of the left ventricle where it can exceed intraventricular systolic pressure (Dieudonné, 1967). This gradient in tissue pressure in the left ventricular wall might account for regional differences in coronary blood flow ; the deep part of the myocardium receiving less flow would therefore be the most predisposed site to myocardial ischemia and anaerobic metabolism (Griggs et al., 1969 ; Gorlin, 1971 ; Lammerant, 1972). Although a lower subendocardial flow has been observed during myocardial ischemia, there is no agreement on whether the intramyocardial flow is uniform or not under normal conditions (Griggs et al., 1972).

3. Neural and neurohumoral factors.

Stimulation of the cardiac sympathetic nerves or infusion of catecholamines elicits a transient increase in the coronary vascular resistance which demonstrates

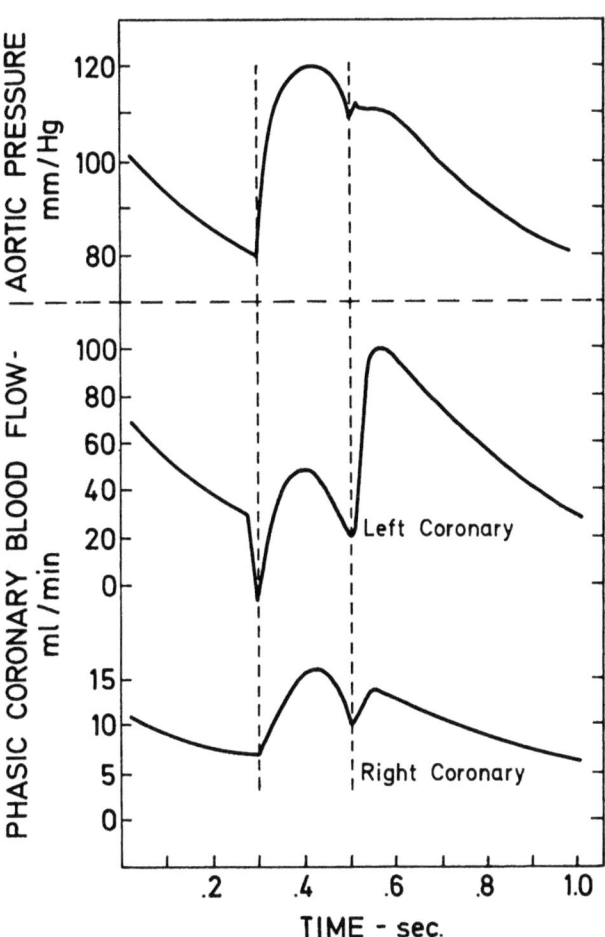

Fig. 3. — Phasic variations in right and left coronary blood flow (from Berne and Levy, 1967).

the existence of neural and neurohumoral control of the coronary blood flow. Both alpha and beta adrenergic receptors are present in the heart but their respective role is still controversial ; vaso-constriction with norepinephrine appears to result from stimulation of alpha receptors while stimulation of beta receptors with isoproterenol would lead to vasodilatation (Gorlin, 1971). Vasoconstriction of the coronary vessels under sympathetic stimulation is rapidly followed however by coronary vasodilatation with a secondary increase in coronary blood flow resulting from the increased metabolic activity of the heart attending sympathetic stimulation (Berne et al., 1965). This diphasic action of the sympathetic nerves on the coronary blood flow illustrates the major role of the local metabolic factors in the control of coronary vascular resistance (Berne et al., 1965 ; Gorlin, 1971). During exercise, for instance, increased sympathetic outflow which tends to constrict the coronary resistance vessels is overruled by local factors and the coronary blood flow increases with no change or only a slight increase in myocardial oxygen extraction (Messer et al., 1962 ; Jorgensen et al., 1971).

Vagal stimulation and acetylcholine administration induce a fall in the coronary vascular resistance ; the role of the vagal system in the control of coronary blood flow appears however to be small (Berne, 1964 ; Feigl, 1969).

B. Determinants of myocardial oxygen consumption.

Experimental investigations in isolated animal heart with separate control of heart rate, pressure and cardiac output have clearly demonstrated that myocardial oxygen consumption is not mainly determined by the external work of the heart but rather by the interplay of three major factors : the intramyocardial tension, the contractile state of the myocardium and the heart rate. Other determinants of $M\dot{V}_{O_2}$ have also been identified but they are of lesser importance : the external work of the heart, the activation energy, and the basal myocardial metabolism (Sonnenblick et al., 1968 ; Braunwald, 1971).

1. Intramyocardial tension.

The pressure developed by the ventricular wall is an essential determinant of $M\dot{V}_{O_2}$ as demonstrated by the close relationship between $M\dot{V}_{O_2}$ and either the tension-time index (Sarnoff et al., 1958) or the product of heart rate and aortic systolic or mean

pressure (Katz and Feinberg, 1958 ; Monroe, 1964). Further studies have indicated that the tension developed in the ventricular wall is a more accurate determinant of $M\dot{V}_{O_2}$ than the pressure generated (Sonnenblick et al., 1968). The intramyocardial tension (T), and consequently $M\dot{V}_{O_2}$, is directly related to the intraventricular pressure (P) and radius (r) and indirectly related to the thickness of the ventricular wall (h) :

$$T = P.r/2h.$$

At fixed values of pressure and wall thickness, an increase in the ventricular volume will consequently result in greater intramyocardial tension and so in greater myocardial oxygen requirements.

The development of tension in the ventricular wall can be defined as the work performed by contractile elements in stretching the elastic components ; it has been termed the internal contractile element work in contrast with the external contractile element work which is performed during muscle shortening against a load (Sonnenblick et al., 1968).

The role of the time during which tension is maintained is still uncertain but Monroe's data (1964) suggest that the development of tension is a far more important determinant of $M\dot{V}_{O_2}$ than the tension maintenance.

2. Contractile state of the myocardium.

The contractile state of the myocardium, which determines the velocity of the contraction, is also very important in the determination of $M\dot{V}_{O_2}$. Sonnenblick et al. (1965) have demonstrated that in the non failing heart, increased myocardial contractility induced by inotropic stimuli caused an increase in $M\dot{V}_{O_2}$ while the tension developed was in fact decreasing. Catecholamines also increase $M\dot{V}_{O_2}$ by a direct stimulating action on myocardial metabolism but this effect is small compared to those of increased velocity of contraction (Braunwald, 1971). The effects of inotropic stimuli on $M\dot{V}_{O_2}$ depend, however, on their associated effect on heart volume, for in the failing heart inotropic agents cause a decrease, not an increase, in $M\dot{V}_{O_2}$ (Covell et al., 1966). This para-doxical action in the failing heart is explained by the decrease of the heart volume due to inotropic agents ; the lower heart volume diminishes the intramyocardial tension and the $M\dot{V}_{O_2}$ to such an extent that the effects on myocardial contractility are masked. The overall effect on $M\dot{V}_{O_2}$ of inotropic stimuli on one hand (Covell et al., 1966) and of drugs decreasing myocardial contractility on the other hand (Graham et al., 1967) will therefore always be determined by the balance between the effects on myocardial contractility and those on heart volume.

3. Heart rate.

The effect of the heart rate on $M\dot{V}_{O_2}$ is obvious since it determines the frequency at which the myocardial wall is stressed. Heart rate has a more complex effect on $M\dot{V}_{O_2}$, however, for it has indeed been demonstrated that the variations in heart rate are associated with changes in myocardial contractility. Increased $M\dot{V}_{O_2}$ with higher heart rate is therefore caused not only by an increase in the total tension developed but also by an increase in myocardial contractility (Boerth et al., 1969). This observation probably helps to explain why indices which do not account for changes in the contractile state of the myocardium but include heart rate were so well related to $M\dot{V}_{O_2}$ (Katz and Feinberg, 1958 ; Sarnoff et al., 1958 ; Monroe, 1964).

4. Other factors.

Basal or resting myocardial metabolism refers to the oxygen needed to sustain the viability of the myocardial cells and represents a small fraction of the total $M\dot{V}_{O_2}$. Although not unsignificant, this portion of $M\dot{V}_{O_2}$ probably corresponds to a relatively stable value (Braunwald, 1971). The activation energy includes the energy required by electrical depolarisation, chemical activation and maintenance of the active state ; the oxygen cost of the activation energy process appears to be small (Braunwald, 1971). The external work of the heart or external contractile element work is that performed when muscle shortens against a load ; the shortening of the myocardium requires oxygen but this factor is of lesser importance than the three major factors cited above (Coleman, 1969).

The free fatty acids (FFA) also influence $M\dot{V}_{O_2}$; increased myocardial uptake of FFA is associated with augmented $M\dot{V}_{O_2}$ despite unchanged mechanical activity (Mjös, 1971). A significant portion of the increased $M\dot{V}_{O_2}$ after infusion of isoproterenol is due to the concomitant increase in arterial FFA concentration and FFA myocardial uptake (Mjös and Kjekshus, 1971). The effects of catecholamines on $M\dot{V}_{O_2}$ are therefore complex and partly due to their lipolytic activity.

5. Indices reflecting myocardial oxygen requirements.

Several indices are used in clinical practice to estimate the myocardial oxygen requirements. Due to the complexity of the factors determing $M\dot{V}_{O_2}$, these indices allow only an approximation of the energy requirements of the myocardium.

Most of these indices are based on the factors which influence the intramyocardial tension and are easily measured, namely the developed pressure, the heart rate and the ejection time. The tension-time index described by Sarnoff et al. (1958) corresponds to the area below the left ventricular pressure curve ; it can also be calculated, with a small error, from the aortic pressure curve as the product of mean systolic aortic pressure and ejection time. Since the time during which tension is maintained does not seem to be a major factor in the determination of $M\dot{V}_{O_2}$, Monroe (1964) proposed to use the product of peak systolic ventricular pressure and heart rate as an index of $M\dot{V}_{O_2}$. A recent study on normal subjects has demonstrated that during exercise $M\dot{V}_{O_2}$ was closely correlated ($r = 0,87$) with the product of heart rate and systolic central blood pressure (Kitamura et al., 1971). This index has also been used by Robinson B. (1967), but he introduced a correction factor for the variations in ejection time ; the product of heart rate, systolic blood pressure and ejection time is also designated as the triple product. Katz and Feinberg (1958) have shown that the product of the mean aortic blood pressure and the heart rate was a reliable index of $M\dot{V}_{O_2}$.

It should be recalled that the pressure wave is increasingly distorted when progressing from the aorta to the peripheral arteries : the systolic blood pressure is indeed higher in the periphery and this difference is enhanced during exercise (Kroeker and Wood, 1955 ; Rowell et al., 1968). Therefore, when systolic blood pressure is used to estimate $M\dot{V}_{O_2}$, it should be measured in the aorta ; this does not apply to mean blood pressure since aortic and peripheral mean blood pressure are very similar (Rowell et al., 1968).

The weakness of all the above indices lies in the fact that they do not take account of other important determinants of $M\dot{V}_{O_2}$, such as the left ventricular volume and the contractile state of the myocardium. On the other hand, these two factors are very difficult to measure directly in humans, particularly during exercise. Changes in myocardial contractility can be estimated by measuring the changes in the peak rate of development of ventricular pressure (dP/dt

max); such measurements have been very useful in the elucidation of the role of myocardial contractility in animal experiments, but they require catheterization of the left ventricle. The mean systolic ejection rate, which is the ratio of stroke volume and ejection time, is often used clinically to estimate the changes in myocardial contractility. The mean systolic ejection rate is however determined not only by the velocity of contraction but also by the ventricular volume : at constant velocity, an increase in volume will indeed determine an increase in mean systolic ejection rate (Levine et al., 1962).

Despite their limitations, the indices of $M\dot{V}_{O_2}$ based on heart rate, systolic or mean pressure, and possibly ejection time are very useful tools in clinical research and they have assisted a great development of our understanding of the pathophysiology of ischemic heart disease.

CHAPTER II

Exercise electrocardiography

The most common indication of exercise testing is the detection of electrocardiographic signs of myocardial ischemia. With the development of multistage exercise tests in recent years, this purpose can now be combined with the determination of functional capacity; this particular aspect will be developed in chapter 3.

Exercise electrocardiography has been used in the diagnosis of coronary heart disease for many years and its validity is now well documented. Epidemiological studies have also indicated the value of exercise electrocardiogram in the detection of latent or subclinical coronary heart disease and in the prediction of the risk of future coronary attacks.

Since the major purpose of exercise electrocardiography is to stress the myocardium in order to provoke electrocardiographic abnormalities indicative of myocardial ischemia, it is essential to examine first the pathophysiological mechanisms underlying the electrocardiographic response. The methods used in exercise electrocardiography are not yet standardized and there is still some discussion concerning the criteria to be used. These methodological problems will be briefly reviewed before we describe the results of this method in patients with documented or silent coronary heart disease. Lastly the electrocardiographic response to exercise can be modified by several therapeutical interventions, and these will be discussed.

The problems of exercise electrocardiography have often been reviewed by eminent specialists. Most recent reviews are those by Bruce and Hornsten (1969), Simonson (1970) and Blomqvist (1971); the book entitled « Measurements in exercise electrocardiography », edited in 1969 by Blackburn, also contains many good papers on a number of aspects of exercise electrocardiography.

PATHOPHYSIOLOGY OF ISCHEMIC ELECTROCARDIOGRAPHIC CHANGES WITH EXERCISE

Among the criteria used in exercise electrocardiography the most reliable sign of myocardial ischemia is undoubtedly the exertional or postexertional horizontal depression of the ST segment. The use of this criterion as a sign of myocardial ischemia is based on extensive clinical research studies which have indicated a good correlation between the occurrence of this abnormality and the presence of clinical coronary heart disease, the risk of future coronary events and the presence of anatomic lesions on the coronary arteries. The degree of ST segment depression is also important since greater depression of the ST segment is attended by a greater risk of coronary attacks and more extensive lesions of the coronary arteries.

The determinants of the ST segment response to exercise can be schematically divided into hemodynamic and metabolic determinants.

A. Hemodynamic determinants.

Myocardial ischemia occurs when the myocardial oxygen requirements are greater than the oxygen supply to the myocardium. In a given patient, angina pectoris, the best clinical symptom of myocardial hypoxia, occurs at a critical level of myocardial oxygen requirements as reflected by the reproducible relationship between the angina threshold and the pressure-rate product (Robinson B., 1967). Like angina pectoris, exercise ST segment depression is also related in most patients to the myocardial oxygen requirements estimated from indices taking account of aortic pressure, heart rate and ejection time (Detry et al., 1970). A given level of ST segment depression during exercise occurs indeed at a reproducible value of the myocardial oxygen requirements (Detry et al., 1970); during atrial pacing ST segment changes also appear at a reproducible heart rate (Lau et al., 1968).

When multistage exercise of increasing severity is prolonged after the onset of a significant ST segment depression, there is also in most patients a close relationship between the magnitude of the ST segment depression and the indices of myocardial oxygen requirements (fig. 4); a linear relationship of this type was present in 12 of 13 patients studied (Detry et al., 1970 ; Detry and Bruce, 1971b). It appears, therefore, that in a given patient the magnitude of ST segment depression during exercise is directly related to the degree of myocardial ischemia. In other words, the amount of ST segment depression during exercise is not a random phenomenon but is related in each subject to the importance of the

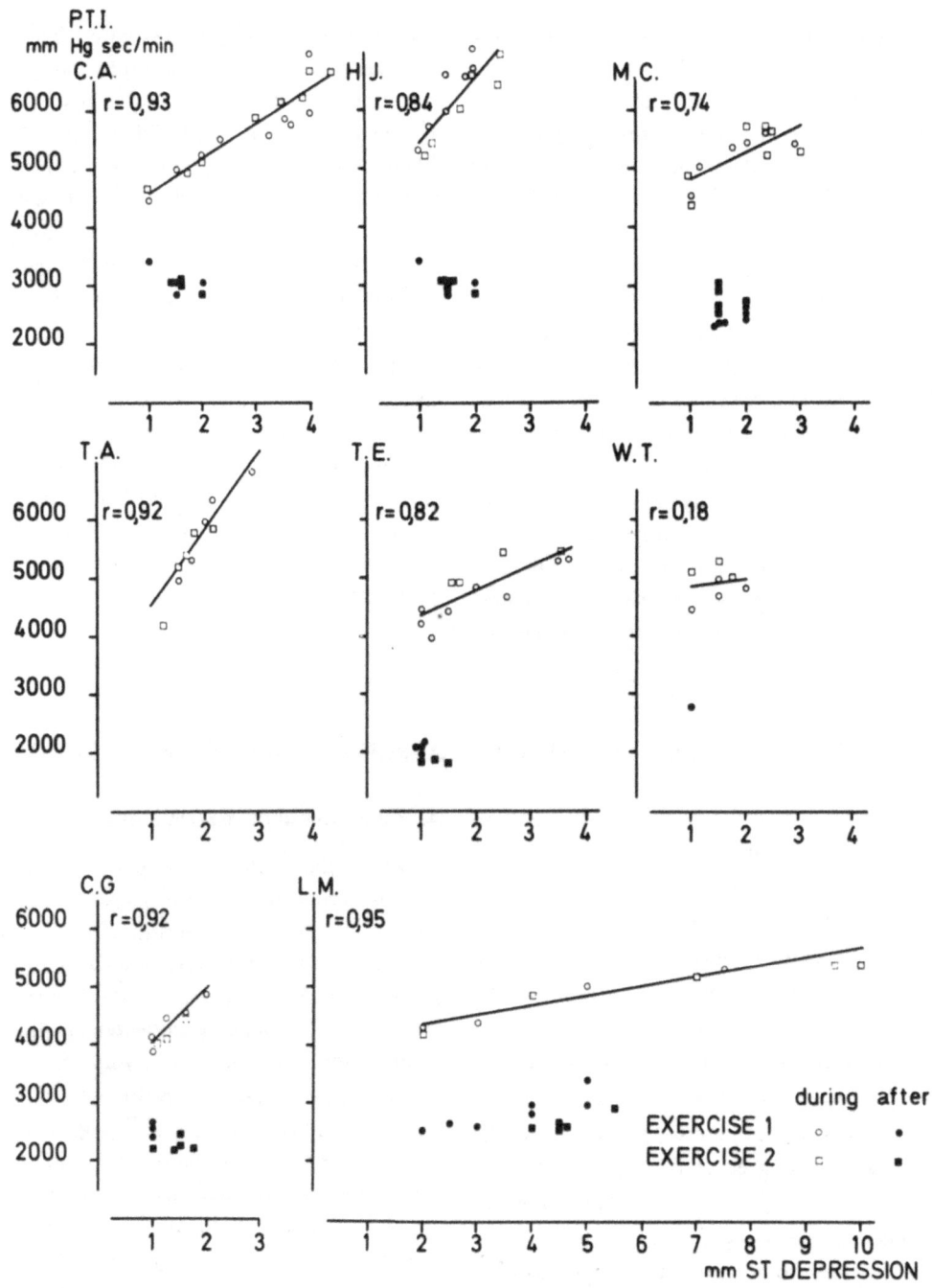

Fig. 4. — Relationship between pressure-time index (PTI) and magnitude of ST segment depression during exercise (open symbols) and recovery (filled-in symbols) in eight subjects. Data collected during two exercises (circles and squares) separated by half an hour of rest. The r values express the correlation between PTI and ST depression during both exercises; this relationship is close except in subject W.T. Note the absence of such relationship during recovery (reprinted from Detry et al., 1970, with the permission of the American Heart Association).

stress applied to the myocardium. During exercise, heart rate alone is closely related to the importance of ST segment depression, which justifies the use of heart rate as a basis for standardizing exercise tests (Detry et al., 1970); the role of the other determinants of the ST segment response should in no case be overlooked, however, since drugs such as nitroglycerin, for instance, modify the relationship between heart rate and ST segment response (Detry and Bruce, 1971a).

The slope of the relationship between the importance of the ST segment depression during exercise and its hemodynamic determinants, as well as the intercept of the slope with the Y axis, vary from subject to subject (fig. 4). The intercept, or the myocardial oxygen requirements at which a significant depression of the ST segment occurs, reflects the coronary reserve : interindividual differences in this value may result from differences in the severity of coronary heart disease and from differences in heart volume or myocardial contractility during exercise (Detry et al., 1970). Interindividual differences in the slope of these relationships also result likely from differences in the severity and/or the extent of coronary lesions.

During recovery from exercise, there is no relationship between the magnitude of the ST segment depression and the hemodynamic determinants of the myocardial oxygen requirements (Detry et al., 1970); also the electrocardiographic aspect often changes during the recovery with the appearance of downsloping ST segment with an inverted T wave (fig. 5). Similarly, after the Master two-step test, there was no correlation between the pressure-time index and electrocardiographic observations (Makous et al., 1964 ; 1969). The mechanisms involved in the postexertional ST response are not well understood; clinical experience as well as the results of epidemiological studies indicate clearly, however, that postexer-

tional ST segment depression also reflects impaired coronary circulation.

Usually the depression of the ST segment is maximal during the last minute of exercise, and during recovery it comes back slowly toward control values. The amount of ST segment depression during recovery, and its duration, appear to depend on the importance of the depression of the ST segment at maximal exercise, for when the latter is increased, as after physical training of angina patients, or decreased with sublingual nitroglycerin, the magnitude of the postexertional ST segment depression and its duration vary accordingly (Detry and Bruce, 1971a; 1971b). These observations suggest that postexertional ECG response is only an indirect consequence of the myocardial ischemia precipitated by exercise, the latter being of course maximum at the maximal exercise level. Other data suggest, however, that ST segment depression occuring after maximal upright exercise may be partly due to a sudden and disproportionate decrease in cardiac output and coronary perfusion pressure when maximal exercise is followed by complete rest in sitting posture (Gutman et al., 1970). These authors have indeed demonstrated that when maximal exercise was followed by walking at a slow speed and at 0° grade for 2 minutes to prevent peripheral venous pooling and sudden decrease in aortic pressure, the maximal postexertional ST segment depression was delayed until the third to fourth minute of the recovery ; unfortunately, this paper does not include data on ECG changes during submaximal and maximal exercise (Gutman et al., 1970). This phenomenon, i.e. inadequate coronary blood flow at lower myocardial oxygen requirements as a consequence of an increase in peripheral venous volume during upright recovery, may partly account for the postexercise ischemic ST depression. The electrocardiograms after the Master two-step test are usually recorded while the patient is lying

V_5

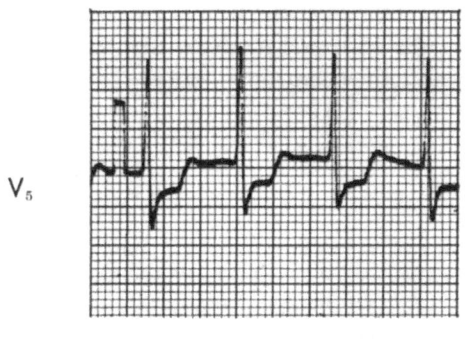 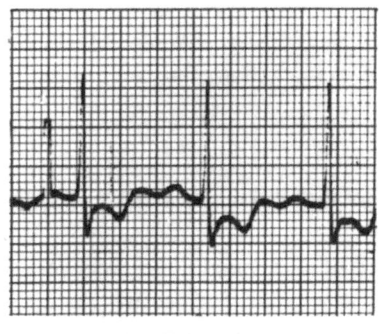

DURING EXERCISE   AFTER EXERCISE

Fig. 5. — Horizontal depression of the ST segment recorded during exercise (left panel) followed by a downsloping ST segment depression with inversion of the T wave during the recovery (right panel).

down: changes in left ventricular volume with postural changes should also be considered as possible determinants of the ECG response after the Master test (Makous et al. 1964).

B. Metabolic factors.

Under normal conditions, the myocardial metabolism is almost exclusively aerobic and lactic acid is extracted by the myocardium to be oxydized (Scheuer, 1967 ; Neill, 1968). During myocardial hypoxia, anaerobic glycolysis of glycogen and glucose leads to the production of lactate which is released in the coronary venous blood. When myocardial ischemia is induced in animals by decreasing the coronary blood flow or in humans by atrial pacing, the extraction of lactate by the myocardium is progressively reduced and finally net production of lactate occurs. The decrease of total lactate extraction probably reflects a balance between zones where the metabolism is normal and zones where lactate production is present (Herman et al., 1967); the subendocardial regions are indeed more sensitive to myocardial hypoxia and to lactate production (Leunissen et al., 1966). Simultaneously with the onset of anaerobic metabolism, there is a release of potassium which is related to the lactate production : 1 mEq of potassium is lost for each 2 millimoles of lactate produced (Case et al., 1969 ; Parker et al., 1969b). The release of potassium and the lactate production are temporarily closely related to other modifications, namely an increase in the left atrial pressure and the appearance of electrocardiographic abnormalities. Case et al. (1969) have demonstrated in dogs that the first electrocardiographic sign of myocardial ischemia was a depression of the J point while horizontal depression of the ST segment appeared later when ischemia was more pronounced.

Both in animals and humans the importance of the horizontal ST segment depression increases with the degree of myocardial anaerobic metabolism (Case et al., 1966, 1969 ; Parker et al., 1969b, 1970b). The correlation between these two parameters is not perfect, however, since the ST segment depression remained unchanged or even decreased when lactate production was still increasing (Parker et al., 1969b); furthermore, lactate production induced by atrial pacing in coronary patients is not always attended by a significant depression of the ST segment (Herman et al., 1967 ; Helfant et al., 1970).

During recovery from these stresses the electrocardiogram returns slowly to control while lactate production progressively disappears : these two phenomena are temporarily related (Parker et al., 1969b). The loss of potassium by the myocardium during atrial pacing is promptly replaced by a net uptake of potassium when the pacing is interrupted (Parker et al., 1970b). During recovery from atrial pacing, therefore, there is no longer a relationship between the loss of potassium and the lactate production, and this apparent lactate production may simply result from the washout of accumulated lactate in the myocardium rather than from persistent anaerobic glycolysis in some regions of the myocardium. Restoration of coronary blood flow to or above control value after myocardial hypoxia in dogs does not cause immediate cessation of lactate production or prompt return of electrocardiogram to control aspect, which indicates that the intramyocardial P_{O_2} is not directly related to the electrocardiographic abnormalities (Case et al., 1966, 1969).

No metabolic factor has yet been identified which could give a satisfactory explanation for the exertional and postexertional ST segment depression. Potassium had been suggested as being directly related to the ST segment depression during myocardial ischemia (Case et al., 1966, 1969 ; Roselle et al., 1966) but this agent cannot account for the post pacing ST segment depression (Parker et al., 1970b); on the other hand lactate production, which is only a reflection of myocardial hypoxia, does not appear to be the causal factor. Ischemic ST segment depression may also very well be under the control of several metabolic factors, some still to be discovered, as there is strong suspicion that myocardial hypoxia is attended by complex metabolic and ionic disturbances.

METHODS IN EXERCISE ELECTROCARDIOGRAPHY

Many methods are used in exercise electrocardiography and they differ especially in the type of exercise test and in the technique for recording the electrocardiogram. These differences are of importance since the choice of the testing procedure largely determines the meaning of the data collected. Efforts to standardize the methods in exercise electrocardiography should therefore be sustained in order to permit comparison of the results of different studies. Standardization will, however, always be limited by pratical considerations such as the time needed to perform the test and the equipment required ; while these problems are of less importance for diagnostic studies performed in well-equipped laboratories, they become crucial in epidemiological studies on large populations.

A. Type of exercise test.

Exercise tests can be divided into single-stage and multistage tests ; the latter are intermittent or continuous, submaximal or maximal.

1. Single-stage tests.

The Master's two-step test, which is well known to all physicians, is a single load test (Master et al., 1942 ; Master 1968). The exercise consists of walking up and down two steps for 1.5 minute (simple test) or 3 minutes (double test); the number of trips required from each subject varies according to age, sex and weight. The energy requirements of the double Master's test is between 1.5 and 1.7 liters of O_2 per minute (Ford and Hellerstein, 1957 ; Rowell et al., 1965). The correction for the body weight equalizes the absolute rather than the relative oxygen cost ; the oxygen cost per kilogram of body weight will therefore be higher for light subjects than for heavy subjects (Rowell et al., 1965).

The major disadvantage of the double Master's test and of other single load tests is their lack of standardization based on myocardial oxygen requirements. The great variability of the relative work load imposed by single-stage tests results in a wide range of heart rate responses ; the peak heart rate during the double step test varied between 105 and 192 beats/minute (Sheffield et al., 1965) and a similar range was reported after a single load treadmill test (Taylor et al., 1969). The stress to the myocardium is therefore negligible in some well - trained subjects while others are tested up to their maximal limits ; the latter is particularly true for many patients with angina pectoris. In addition, the double Master's test provides only a low incidence of positive electrocardiographic findings in patients with documented coronary heart disease.

The double Master's test has, however, been used in many clinical studies which have provided very useful information. Since it is simple to perform, it may still be used as a screening procedure ; the heart rate response should always be taken into account, however, in interpreting the electrocardiographic response to this test.

2. Multistage test.

Multistage tests are now recommended since they do not present the limitations of single load tests. The intensity of the exercise and its end-point are adjusted to each patient's capacity, so that the stress to the myocardium is similar for all subjects. Relative severity of the exercise is judged from the heart rate response ; the test is started at a low level and its intensity is then gradually increased up to a predetermined submaximal heart rate or up to the maximal heart rate. The heart rate represents an excellent basis for standardization of electrocardiographic exercise tests since it is a major determinant of the myocardial oxygen requirements and of the ST segment response to exercise (Detry et al., 1970). Multistage near-maximal or maximal tests provide greater diagnostic sensitivity than single load exercise tests ; another important advantage of multistage tests is the measurement of physical capacity (see chapter 3).

Many multistage exercise tests are now in use and their characteristics have been recently reviewed (Taylor et al., 1969). As long as the heart rate is taken into account, the choice of the ergometer is not critical and the step test, the biccycle ergometer or the treadmill can be used. Some authors use several work loads separated by rest periods while others prefer an uninterrupted multistage test : the intervening rest periods prolong the duration of the test but they also provide data during recovery at low exercise levels. The end-point of the test may be predetermined - the exercise is stopped when a target heart rate has been reached (submaximal or near-maximal testing) - or the subject is asked to exercise up to his maximal limits.

The target heart rate (table 2) is usually 80 to 90 % of the maximal heart rate ; due to differences

TABLE 2

Target heart rate (beats/minute) in multistage exercise tests.

Age group	Lester et al. (1967, 1968)*	Scandinavian Committee (1967)
20 - 29	175	170
30 - 39	170	160
40 - 49	166	150
50 - 59	162	140
60 - 69	158	130

* These values correspond to 90 % of the predicted maximal heart rate.

in observed maximal heart rate, the values recommended by Lester et al. (1967, 1968) are higher than those of a Scandinavian committee (1967). Others do not take into account the decrease of maximal heart rate with age and test their subjects up to an absolute heart rate between 150 and 170 (Sjöstrand, 1947; Hellerstein and Hornsten, 1966; Messin et al., 1966). The choice of a submaximal or nearmaximal heart rate as the target is based partly on the fear to exercise subjects to the maximal level; Lester et al. (1967) have indeed reported that potentially dangerous ventricular arrhythmias were more likely to occur between 90 and 100 % of the maximal heart rate.

The predicted maximal heart rate used in the estimation of the relative severity of the exercise is questionable, however, since there is no agreement between the published data (fig. 6); for instance,

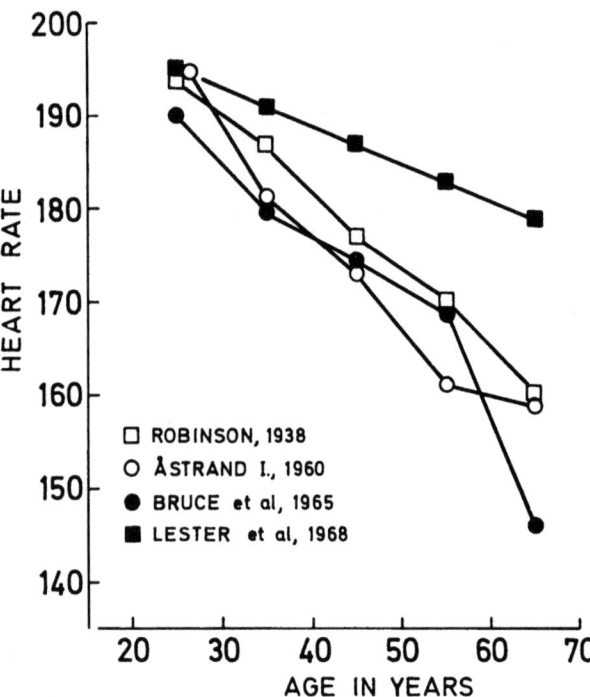

Fig. 6. — Influence of age on the maximal heart rate of healthy men.

In multistage maximal exercise tests, the subject is asked to push himself to his maximal limits; in the absence of untoward events at submaximal exercise levels, the intensity of the exercise is increased until the subject or patient can no longer continue. The end-point of the test is therefore not arbitrarily fixed as in submaximal or nearmaximal exercise tests, but should represent the maximal working capacity of the subject. The maximal tests provide a higher incidence of positive electrocardiographic findings and the physical work capacity of the subject can be measured. The reason for stopping the test may be the unwillingness of the subject to go further, the occurrence of symptoms such as dyspnea, hypotension, fatigue or angina pectoris, or the fact that the subject has reached his true maximal oxygen intake; therefore, these maximal exercise tests do not always provide a measurement of the maximal oxygen intake.

Bruce's multistage treadmill test (Bruce et al., 1963; Doan et al., 1965) includes 7 levels of exercise of increasing severity; each stage lasts 3 minutes and the intensity of the exercise is increased every 3 minutes, without interruption of the test, by changing both the grade and the speed of the treadmill (table 3). With this procedure it is possible to test both limited patients and trained athletes according to the same protocol and in a short time.

TABLE 3

Characteristics of Bruce's multistage treadmill test (from Bruce et al., 1963 and Doan et al., 1966).

Stage *	Speed (miles per hour)	Grade %
1	1.7	10
2	2.5	12
3	3.4	14
4	4.2	16
5	5.0	18
6	5.5	20
7	6.0	22

* Duration of each stage is 3 minutes.

B. Technical aspects. Leads systems.

Interpretation of electrocardiographic response to exercise depends greatly on the quality of the records submitted for analysis; the amount of data collected is also important since increasing the number of

the mean maximal heart rate in the 50 - 59 age group varies from 183 (Lester et al., 1968) to 161 (Åstrand, 1960). Furthermore, the standard deviation of these mean maximal heart rate values is important, approximately 10 beats. If all the reported data were real maximal heart rates, the range would be so great that the mean maximal values would be of little physiological significance.

leads recorded, for instance, and recording the electrocardiogram during exercise, enhance the diagnostic sensitivity of exercise electrocardiography. The technological and procedural aspect of exercise electrocardiography have recently been reviewed in detail by Blackburn (1969).

A basic requirement of all systems is a good contact between skin and electrodes. The skin should be carefully prepared to decrease its resistance and the horny layer of epidermis has to be eliminated. The use of light silver electrodes filled with special electrode jelly and properly fixed on the skin provides a stable skin-electrode contact, thus avoiding artefacts due to motion ; the development of small flexible ECG cables also helps to improve the quality of the records (Blackburn, 1969 ; Blomqvist, 1971).

Three ECG leads systems are used, i.e. the conventional 12 leads system, bipolar chest leads and the orthogonal 3 leads systems.

Conventional ECG 12 leads systems are widely used to record the electrocardiogram in supine posture after the double-step test and the major part of our knowledge of exercise electrocardiography is derived from this system. To permit the use of a 12 leads system during exercise, Mason and Likar (1966) proposed fixing the remote limbs electrodes on the torso ; this modification does not significantly alter the amplitude of the ECG complex in the standard leads and provides good records during exercise. The information provided by the conventional or modified 12 leads system is redundant ; Blackburn and Katigbak (1964) have in fact reported that virtually all the ST-T information of postexertional records is contained in 6 of the 12 leads (D_2, aV_F, V_3, V_4, V_5 and V_6) while most (89 %) of the information is found in V_5 alone. Among 56 angina patients exhibiting a positive ST response during or after a multistage exercise test, however, 19 (34 %) had positive findings in only one lead ; of these 19 patients only 2 had a positive response in V_5, while 7 had isolated positive findings in V_6, 4 in V_4, and 2 in V_3, D_2 or D_3 (Mason et al., 1967). In the above mentioned study, the use of the V_5 lead alone would give a high proportion of false negative responses, at least 30 %. The proportion of patients exhibiting diagnostic findings in vertically oriented leads can be as high as 45 % (Mason et al., 1967) and these findings are isolated, i.e. absent in V_3, V_4, V_5 and V_6, in approximately 10 % of the patients (Blackburn and Katigbak, 1964 ; Mason et al., 1967). It is therefore clear that several leads should be recorded during or after exercise : the best combination appears

to be V_3, V_4, V_5, V_6, D_2 and D_3 or aV_F. When exercise is performed in supine position, however, Kassebaum et al. (1968) reported that D_2, D_3 and aV_F were the most sensitive leads.

Many *bipolar leads systems* have been proposed and they differ in the position of the reference electrode ; the exploring electrode is usually placed in C_5 (V_5) which is the most sensitive location for ST depression display (Blackburn et al., 1966). The bipolar lead CM_5 (chest-manubrium) has the greatest sensitivity for detection of ST depression and performs better than the conventional precordial V_5 ; this greater sensitivity of bipolar leads is due chiefly to the greater amplitude of R wave in these leads and also from their more vertical orientation (Blackburn et al., 1966). As with conventional leads, the use of multiple bipolar leads is attended by greater sensitivity. Bipolar leads systems are simpler to use than conventional ECG systems ; if only a single lead is to be used, CM_5 appears best in all respects (Blackburn et al., 1966). The major problem with bipolar chest leads is that their diagnostic power has never been directly established, and in this respect conventional leads appear preferable.

Orthogonal leads XYZ are mainly used in exercise electrocardiography for research purposes. One advantage of Frank leads over conventional 12 leads is a substantial reduction in the amount of data collected without loss of information, which is important for further quantitative analysis of the data (Blomqvist, 1965 ; Bruce et al., 1966); in addition, the orthogonal leads allow a spatial representation of ST vectors. Hornsten and Bruce (1969) have recorded simultaneously during and after maximal exercise the orthogonal XYZ leads and a simple bipolar CB_5 (chest-right scapular); the diagnostic power of the ST forces of the computed bipolar lead was similar to that of the 3 Frank leads ; they concluded that for practical purposes, classification of ST responses was as reliable with a simple bipolar lead than with the more comprehensive Frank leads.

Electrocardiogram should be recorded not only after an exercise test but also during the exercise itself ; this will increase the safety of the procedure and also the diagnostic sensitivity of the test. Mason et al. (1967) have demonstrated that with the double step test, 5 % of the patients exhibited abnormal ST responses only during exercise ; with multistage tests, this percentage was 9 %. Similar observations have been made by Bellet et al. (1962) and Goenen et al. (1970). It is also essential that comparisons should be based only on electrocardiograms recorded in the same posture. With bicycle or treadmill exercise tests, an ECG should therefore always be recorded in the sitting position before the test ; this procedure may also be helpful in revealing ECG orthostatic changes.

C. Risks of exercise testing. Precautions.

Rochmis and Blackburn (1971) have recently analyzed the morbidity and mortality attributable to exercise testing in a large sample of 170.000 tests performed in 73 centers ; most (66 %) of these tests were multistage progressive tests. Sixteen deaths (1/10.000) were attributed to the exercise tests ; 8 of these deaths occurred within an hour of the test, 4 within a day and 4 within a week. The mortality was not related to the intensity of the exercise test since 10 deaths occurred after near-maximal or maximal tests and 6 after submaximal tests ; in half of the cases (5/10) attributed to maximal exercise testing, the test had in fact been interrupted at a low exercise level. In 4 of the cases reported by Rochmis and Blackburn (1971) the relationship between exercise testing and death is questionable since the test was completed without any problem and the patients developed an acute myocardial infarction several hours to several days later. In one case, the test was inadvertently performed in the presence of an acute myocardial infarction without physician screening. This low mortality rate in exercise testing (in fact less than 1/10.000) probably accounts for the absence of death in smaller samples previously reported

(Ellestad et al., 1969 ; Bruce, 1970 ; Rousseau and Brasseur, 1972).

In the same study, a further 40 subjects had to be hospitalized after the exercise test for non fatal events, which gives a morbidity rate of 2.4/10.000 ; the exact reason for these short term hospitalizations was not reported (Rochmis and Blackburn, 1971). Other authors have reported rare instances of non-fatal myocardial infarction or ventricular fibrillation after exercise testing (Bruce et al., 1968 ; Ellestad et al., 1969 ; Bruce, 1970 ; Rousseau and Brasseur, 1972).

Several precautions should be taken for exercise testing. The patient's history sould always be taken, and a physical examination and resting electrocardiogram should always be performed before the test. Contraindications to exercise testing include a recent myocardial infarction (less than 2 months), a recent worsening of angina pectoris and acute non cardiac illnesses ; recent history of syncopal episodes, or serious arrythmias represent relative contraindications. The exercise test should always be supervised by a well trained physician and resuscitation equipment should be at hand. Constant oscilloscopic monitoring of the electrocardiogram during exercise and initial recovery undoubtedly increases the safety of the procedure. The physician should also be prepared to interrupt the test on account of one of the following signs or symptoms : occurrence of 3 or more consecutive premature ventricular beats, onset of an ataxic gait, or progressive hypotension (Bruce and Hornsten, 1969 ; Rochmis and Blackburn, 1971).

CRITERIA FOR INTERPRETATION

In order to be taken as reflecting myocardial ischemia, an electrocardiographic criterion should be both sensitive and specific ; specificity means that it is rarely or never demonstrated by normal subjects while sensitivity requires that it is exhibited by many and ideally all patients with coronary artery disease. Since there is no perfect criterion for electrocardiographic ischemia, the choice of criteria will inevitably depend on a balance between the requirements for specificity and those for sensitivity. While numerous criteria for ischemic electrocardiographic response have been proposed in the past, the results of long term follow-up studies and those of anatomo-electrical comparisons permit a simpler definition of the criteria to be used.

A. Ischemic ST depression.

The term « ischemic ST depression », introduced by Wood et al. in 1950, refers to an horizontal or downsloping depression of the ST segment (fig. 5) ; the ischemic depression of the ST segment is the most commonly accepted electrocardiographic criterion for diagnosis of coronary insufficiency. This abnormality is extremely rare in young healthy subjects, even after maximal exercise (Doan et al., 1965 ; Bellet and Roman, 1967). This criterion has been validated by many follow-up studies which have indicated a significantly higher mortality due to coronary disease in the subjects exhibiting ischemic ST depression $\geqslant 0.5$ mm (Brody, 1959 ; Mattingly, 1962 ; Rumball and Acheson, 1963 ; Robb and Marks, 1964 ; Bellet et al., 1967 ; Punsar et al., 1968 ; Åstrand and Lundman, 1968 ; Doyle and Kinch, 1970) ; the risk of future coronary events was also directly related to the importance of the ischemic ST depression. Lastly, we have demonstrated that the onset of a significant horizontal depression of the ST segment, and its importance during graded exercise, were directly related to the severity of the stress applied to the myocardium (Detry et al., 1970).

Most authors now require an ischemic ST depression $\geqslant$ 1 mm in order to consider the response to be abnormal (Wood et al., 1950 ; Mason et al., 1967 ; Harrison and Reeves, 1968 ; Blomqvist, 1971) ; if an ST segment depression $\geqslant$ 0.5 mm is considered abnormal, as still suggested by Master (1968), the percentage of false positive diagnoses increases to unacceptable values (Friedberg et al., 1962 ; Mason et al., 1967 ; McConahay et al., 1971). Recently Goenen et al. (1970) required an horizontal depression of the ST segment $\geqslant$ 2 mm and surprisingly the sensitivity of the exercise test remained good, while, Friedberg et al. (1962), using the same criterion, reported a sharp decrease in sensitivity.

B. Slowly ascending ST depression.

The significance of a depression of the J point followed by an upsloping ST segment is still a matter for discussion. While many authors consider that the depression of the J point is a normal response to exercise (Wood et al., 1950 ; Mattingly, 1962 ; Rumball and Acheson, 1963 ; Robb and Marks, 1964 ; Mason et al., 1967 ; Blackburn et al., 1970), others regard important depression of the J point ($\geqslant$ 2 mm) as a suspicious response (Harrison and Reeves, 1968). Punsar et al. (1968) made an important contribution to this problem by separating the ST depression with slowly ascending ST segment - S type, which does not reach base line before T wave - from the ST depression with rapidly ascending ST segment - R type, which traverses the baseline before T wave - (fig. 7) ; in a follow-up study of 1534 men, they demonstrated that ST depressions of S type were associated with a greater subsequent incidence of coronary disease, while ST depression of R type had no pejorative prognostic significance. Brody and Springs had already reported in 1959 that important depression of the J point ($\geqslant$ 1.5 mm) were attended by a worse prognostic, but unfortunately they did not separate the J depression into S and R types.

Bruce now regards any postexertional ST segment depression $\geqslant$ 1 mm, lasting for 0.06 sec at least, as an abnormal response, whether horizontal, upsloping or downsloping (Bruce and Hornsten, 1969) ; in fact, upsloping ST depression of 1 mm, 0.06 sec after the nadir of the S wave, often represents a slow upsloping ST depression of the S type. This type of ST depression often precedes a true ischemic depression and may be sometimes recorded in one lead while another records a true ischemic aspect (Russek, 1957 ; Bruce and Hornsten, 1969) ; in addition, early myocardial ischemia in dogs is accompanied by a depression of the J point, simultaneous with the onset of anaerobic metabolism, while the ischemic ST configuration is a later feature (Case et al., 1969). While the exact diagnostic significance of slowly upsloping ST depression has still to be firmly established, several authors using a computer averaging technique of the exercise electrocardiogram consider these responses doubtful or abnormal (McHenry et al., 1968 ; Bruce and Hornsten, 1969 ; Sheffield et al., 1969).

C. ST segment elevation.

Elevation of the ST segment induced by exercise is often considered a criterion of myocardial ischemia ; Master (1968, 1970) requires an ST segment eleva-

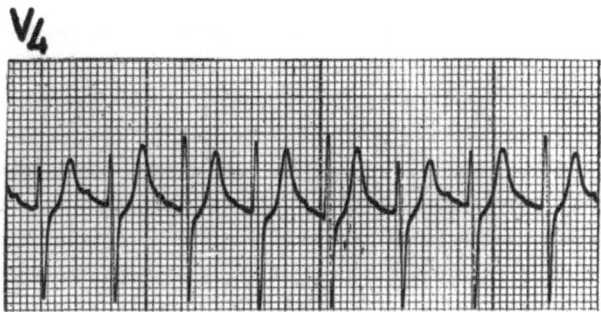

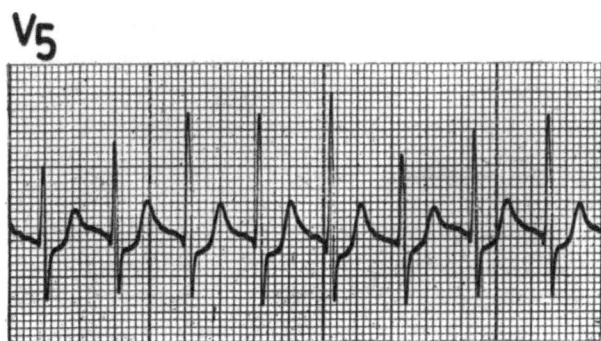

Fig. 7. — ECG recorded after exercise. The lead V_4 exhibits a rapidly ascending ST segment depression (R type) while V_5 exhibits a slowly ascending ST segment depression (S type).

tion of 0,5 mm in order to consider the response as abnormal while others require 1 mm (Mason et al., 1967 ; Fortuin and Friesinger, 1970). This type of response to exercise, although rare, may reflect a more severe degree of myocardial ischemia than does ST segment depression. In experimental myocardial ischemia caused by coronary ligation in the dog, ST elevation is indeed recorded in the most ischemic part of the ventricle while regions with less profound ischemia exhibit ST depression (Ekmekci et al., 1961). Among 12 patients developing such ST segment elevation after exercise, 11 had major coronary lesions demonstrated by coronary arteriography and the short-term prognosis of these patients was very poor, since 4 out of 10 patients followed for one year or more had died suddenly (Fortuin and Friesinger, 1970) ; unfortunately these authors did not include left ventriculographic data in their report, but they stated that ventricular aneurysm was not a satisfactory explanation for their findings. Atterhög et al. (1971) have recently reported that ST segment elevation with exercise was often recorded in the leads facing the myocardial infarction a few weeks after acute anterior myocardial infarction, but tended to diseappear progressively when the interval between the acute episode and exercise testing increased.

Many patients with ventricular aneurysm present at rest an elevation of the ST segment in the leads regarding the aneurysm ; when it is not already present at rest, ST segment elevation is often precipitated by exercise (Bruce et al., 1963 ; Gorlin et al., 1967). Whether or not ST elevation with exercise reported by Fortuin and Friesinger (1970) in fact reflects asynergy of the left ventricular contraction with myocardial ischemia (Dwyer, 1970), or has a different significance remains to be established. In any event, appearance of an ST segment elevation with exercise in electrocardiographic leads demonstrating signs of previous myocardial infarction should always produce suspicion that a ventricular akinetic or dyskinetic zone is present, even if otherwise unsuspected.

D. Other criteria.

The criteria initially described by Master et al. (1942) and subsequently refined by Lepeschkin and Surawic (1958) and Master and Rosenfeld (1961) are responsible for a high incidence of positive findings in normal subjects (Unterman and De Graaf, 1948 ; Wood et al., 1950 ; Thomas, 1951 ; Davis et al., 1953 ; Russek, 1957 ; Lepeschkin and Surawic, 1958 ; Friedberg et al., 1962). Among these criteria,

the isolated modification of the T wave, the junctional ST depression of less than 2 mm, the QX/QT and the QT/QTc ratios, the appearance of transient intraventrivular conduction disturbance (right or left bundle branch block) or minor A-V conduction trouble have to be considered normal findings since they were not related to a significantly higher mortality in follow-up studies (Brody and Springs, 1959 ; Mattingly, 1962 ; Rumball and Acheson, 1963 ; Robb and Marks, 1964 ; Blackburn et al., 1970 ; Doyle and Kinch, 1970).

The significance of premature ventricular contractions during or after exercise is not yet fully understood. Premature ventricular contractions at rest or during ordinary daily activity are related to a subsequent higher incidence of coronary artery disease (Hinkle et al., 1969 ; Blackburn et al., 1970); these rhythm disturbances are very common, however, even in a normal population (Hinkle et al., 1969). Appearance of premature ventricular beats after an exercise test is not significantly related to a greater risk of coronary disease (Brody and Springs, 1959 ; Blackburn et al., 1970); furthermore, when exercise testing is repeated after several weeks, rhythm or conduction disturbances are only poorly reproducible (Gooch and McConnel, 1970). Multifocal premature ventricular beats with exercise, although more commonly seen in patients with coronary heart disease (6.7 %), are not rare (2.1 %) in healthy subjects (McHenry et al., 1972). In view of their low specificity and great variability, rhythm disturbances with exercise should not be considered as a criterion of myocardial ischemia. However, the occurrence of 3 or more consecutive premature ventricular contractions is a strict indication for interrupting the testing procedure, on account of the risk of ventricular tachycardia or fibrillation (Bruce and Hornsten, 1969).

E. Observer variation. Need for quantification.

There is great interobserver variation in the interpretation of the electrocardiographic response to exercise. A sample of 38 records was submitted to 14 observers who had to code the tracing as normal, borderline, abnormal or technically unsatisfactory (Blackburn et al., 1968). Complete agreement between all observers was present in only 9 of the 38 records (24 %) while 17 tracings (45 %) were coded as normal by some observers and abnormal by others ; minor disagreement (records coded as abnormal or borderline and borderline or normal by all readers) was noted in 12 tracings (31 %).

The percentage of tracings considered abnormal varied from 5% to 58% of the records analyzed. Intraobserver variation was also considerable, for 8 to 38% of the records were coded differently by the same observer 10 days apart. Principal reasons for these disagreements are the lack of precisely defined criteria, differences in opinion regarding the significance of upsloping ST segment depression, and the poor technical quality of some records. Variability in interpretation is greater for the tracings recorded during exercise (Blackburn et al., 1968); Punsar et al. (1968) also mentioned that recognition of slowly upsloping ST depression was attended by greater interobserver variability than for true ischemic ST depression.

This wide range of variation in interpretation of exercise electrocardiograms clearly indicates the need for more objective and quantitative analysis. Several computer systems are now used to provide quantitative analysis of exercise electrocardiograms and this approach is undergoing constant development. Some principles are basic to nearly all systems, however, and they will be outlined briefly.

The electrocardiogram recorded on magnetic tape during the exercise test is first digitized and averaged, which can be done by means of a small and fairly inexpensive computer. Sampling by the computer should be initiated by a signal which has a constant time relation with the electrocardiographic complex. Since it is essential to refer the ST-T voltage to the PR level of the same beat, the triggering signal has to be anticipated, and this can be done by using a two channels magnetic tape and generating a trigger signal preceding the QRS complex to be sampled (Blomqvist, 1965; Bruce et al., 1966). The ECG signal is fed into a pulse oscillator which generates a number of pulses proportional to the instantaneous amplitude of the analog input signal; the pulses corresponding to a specific sampling period of each cardiac cycle are stored in one of the computer's memories (addresses) where they are added to those previously stored at the same address. The averaging of a signal reduces the noise in proportion to the square root of the number of signals averaged. Bruce et al. (1966) average a constant number of beats (100) while Blomqvist (1965) adjusts the number of beats to the heart rate.

The second step in computer exercise electrocardiography, i.e. the analysis of the data, largely depends on the available computer facilities; sophisticated programs have been developed which permit identification of the ECG waves, amplitude measurements and printed display of the data in numerical or graphical form.

The information so provided by computer averaging has to be reduced to concise and clinically useful information. For ST-T analysis Bruce et al. (1966) have selected fixed interval sampling points while Blomqvist (1965) divides the ST-T segment in 8 subsegments whose duration is consequently determined by the cycle lenth. Sheffield et al. (1969) have recently described a system to quantify the negative ST integral, i.e. the surface of the depressed ST area expressed in microvolt-seconds.

DIAGNOSTIC AND PROGNOSTIC POWER OF EXERCISE ELECTROCARDIOGRAPHY

Many clinical studies have demonstrated the validity of exercise electrocardiography in the diagnosis of coronary artery disease, but in recent years development of coronary arteriography has permitted a better evaluation of the sensitivity and specificity(*) of this diagnostic procedure. The poor prognostic significance of electrocardiographic abnormalities induced by exercise in apparently normal subjects has stimulated efforts from researchers to delimit the syndrome of latent coronary heart disease more satisfactorily, with the hope of developing methods which will adequately prevent its progression to overt disease. Finally, wider application of exercise electrocardiography in patients with non-coronary heart disease raises questions about the significance of the abnormalities often encountered in such patients.

(*) Sensitivity (%) is the ratio of the true positives (abnormal coronary arteriography and abnormal exercise electrocardiogram) to the sum of the true positives and the false negatives (abnormal coronary arteriography and normal electrocardiogram).
Specificity (%) is the ratio of the true negatives (normal coronary arteriography and normal electrocardiogram) to the sum of the true negatives and the false positives (normal coronary arteriography and abnormal exercise electrocardiogram).

A. Documented coronary heart disease.

The sensitivity and specificity of exercise electrocardiography in the diagnosis of coronary heart disease depend on the severity of the criteria used and on the intensity of the exercise test (table 4). It is clear that the sensitivity of exercise electrocardiogram decreases when a more severe criterion is used ; at the same time, however, specificity increases, i.e. the percentage of false positive diagnoses is reduced. This trend is present with the Master's two-step test (McConahay et al., 1971) and with multistage near maximal tests (Mason et al., 1967). The sensitivity of exercise electrocardiogram is also increased by recording the ECG during exercise (Bellet et al., 1962 ; Mason et al., 1967 ; Goenen et al., 1970) and by using multiple leads systems (Bellet et al., 1964 ; Blackburn et al., 1966 ; Mason et al., 1967).

1. Master's double two-step test.

The sensitivity of an ischemic ST segment depression $\geqslant$ 1 mm precipitated by a double Master's two step test can be estimated at 46 %, for this response was present in 79 of 172 (46 %) patients who had a luminal narrowing $\geqslant$ to 50 % of at least one coronary vessel (Demany et al., 1967 ; Most et al., 1969 ; McConahay et al., 1971)(*). In these studies the percentage of false negative electrocardiographic responses was 54 % (93/172); it varied from 65 %

(McConahay et al., 1971) to 42 % (Most et al., 1969). The specificity of the ischemic ST segment depression $\geqslant$ 1 mm after the Master's test has been variously assessed : it was perfect (0 % false positive responses) in 100 subjects studied by McConahay et al. (1971) while Demany et al. (1967) reported 30 % (10/33) false positive responders. Most et al. (1969) did not report electrocardiographic responses of subjects with normal coronary vessels. The results of Demany et al. (1967) are in striking contrast with all other published data (Hultgren et al., 1967) even with maximal exercise testing.

2. Multistage tests.

Multistage near-maximal tests are much more sensitive in the diagnosis of anatomical coronary heart disease (tables 4 and 5); overall sensitivity of an ST segment depression $\geqslant$ 1 mm during or after near-maximal exercise test was 76 % in a sample of 188 patients - table 5 (Mason et al., 1967 ; Kassebaum et al., 1968 ; Roitman et al., 1970). There is no apparent explanation for the lower sensitivity reported by Kassebaum et al. (1968), except perhaps the fact that in this study exercise was performed in supine posture. The specificity of near-maximal exercise testing is satisfactory since the percentage of false positive responders was only 8 % (table 5); in fact, when the clinician is faced with a problem of diagnosis of a chest pain, the proportion of false

TABLE 4

Sensitivity and specificity of ischemic ST segment depression in the diagnosis of anatomical coronary disease. Influence of the importance of the ST segment depression and of the type of exercise test.

Importance of ST segment depression	Type of exercise test			
	Double Master's step test *		Near-maximal exercise test **	
mm	Sensitivity %	Specificity %	Sensitivity %	Specificity %
$\geqslant$ 0.5	63	83	88	69
$\geqslant$ 0.75	42	91	84	83
$\geqslant$ 1.0	35	100	78	89
$\geqslant$ 1.5	26	100	37	100
$\geqslant$ 2.0	20	100	22	100

* From data on 100 patients (McConahay et al., 1971). ** From data on 84 patients (Mason et al., 1967).

(*) The sensitivity of the Master's double step test increases to 77 % (59/77) when a luminal narrowing $\geqslant$ 75 % is required for a true positive diagnosis (Cohn et al., 1971).

TABLE 5

Correlation between coronary arteriography and ischemic ST segment depression $\geq$ 1 mm in near-maximal exercise testing of patients with typical or atypical chest pain.

Source	Number of cases	C + E +	C + E —	C — E +	C — E —	Sensitivity %	Specificity %
Mason et al. (1967)	84	38	11	4	31	78	89
Kassebaum et al. (1968)	68	18	18	1	31	50	97
Roitman et al. (1970)	46	24	6	2	14	80	87
TOTAL	188	80	25	7	76	76	92

C + indicates the presence of coronary stenosis $\geq$ to 50 % of the lumen of at least one coronary vessel and C — the absence of such finding.

E + and E — refer to the presence or the absence of ischemic ST segment depression $\geq$ 1 n.m during or after exercise.

TABLE 6

Correlation between clinical history, electrocardiographic response to near-maximal exercise and coronary arteriographic data in 152 patients (adapted from Mason et al., 1967, and Kassebaum et al., 1968).

Classification of the patients		Coronary arteriography **	
Typical angina pectoris	ECG response to exercise *	C +	C —
+	+	48	1
+	—	20	11
—	+	8	4
—	—	9	51

* Positive(+) ECG response to exercise refers to ST segment depression $\geq$ 1 mm.

** C + and C — (see legend of table 5).

sensitivity and specificity of clinical history on one hand, and near-maximal exertional electrocardiogram on the other hand, in the detection of coronary lesions are compared in a sample of 152 patients - table 6 (Mason et al., 1967 ; Kassebaum et al., 1968). The sensitivity of clinical history (presence or absence of a typical angina pectoris) is greater than that of exertional electrocardiogram (80 % versus 66 %) but its specificity is lower (82 % versus 93 %). Combination of these 2 diagnostic procedures reveals that 98 % (48/49) of the patients with typical angina pectoris and positive electrocardiographic responses have abnormal coronary arteriography while, when atypical chest pain is attended by a normal electrocardiographic response to exercise, the coronary vessels are normal in 85 % of the subjects (51/60). Discrepancy between clinical diagnosis and electrocardiographic data results in frequent misclassification of the patients, for in 35 % (15/43) of these patients, the coronary vessels were normal despite a positive electrocardiographic response to exercise or the existence of a typical chest pain. Discordances between electrocardiographic and clinical findings consequently represent a good indication for coronary arteriography.

3. False negative responses.

Even with near-maximal exercise tests, there is a significant percentage (24 %) of patients with documented anatomical coronary disease who have normal electrocardiographic responses to exercise (table 5). The proportion of false negative responders

positive responders is lower, since only 7 out of 188 patients (3,6 %) presented such response. It has been claimed that the sensitivity of maximal exercise testing was even greater than that of near-maximal testing (Doan et al., 1966 ; Lester et al., 1967); at our best knowledge, however, electrocardiographic data collected with maximal exercise tests have never been systematically compared with the anatomical state of the coronary arteries.

Typical angina pectoris correlates well with the existence of anatomical coronary heart disease. The

tends to be less in patients presenting wide-spread coronary lesions (table 7): the difference is particularly marked when patients with one vessel disease are compared with those having involvement of 2 coronary vessels, but is less clear when patients with 2 and 3 vessels disease are compared. Data from other investigators could not be included in table 7 since they did not classify their patients according to the number of coronary vessels involved (Demany et al., 1967 ; Hultgren et al., 1967 ; Mason et al., 1967 ; Roitman et al., 1970); however, all these authors stated that the sensitivity of exercise electrocardiography was not related to the severity and distribution of the coronary lesions.

The presence of collateral vessels does not seem to influence the electrocardiographic response to exercise since in most studies the incidence of demonstrable collaterals in false negative responders is identical to that in true positive responders (Demany et al., 1967 ; Most et al., 1969 ; Tuna and Amplatz, 1970 ;

McConahay et al., 1971). The coronary collateral vessels develop in response to severe coronary arterial stenosis or obstruction and their frequency is related to the severity of coronary heart disease (Gensini and Da Costa, 1969 ; Sheldon, 1969); they do not appear to prevent the development of an ischemic electrocardiographic response to exercise. Most et al. (1969) even reported a greater frequency of collateral coronary vessels in patients with abnormal postexercise electrocardiogram ; collateral vessels were also more frequent in patients with more important ST depression.

Normal electrocardiographic responses to exercise in presence of a coronary occlusion could also result from complete transformation of the myocardial tissue distal to occlusion into a fibrous scar (Blomqvist, 1971); however, this explanation cannot account for normal exercise electrocardiogram in multiple vessels disease.

TABLE 7

Proportion of false negative electrocardiographic responses to exercise according to the degree of coronary heart disease.

Number of vessels involved *	Incidence of false negative responders **		
	1	2	3
Most et al. (1967) Master test	9/13 (69 %)	6/13 (46 %)	12/27 (31 %)
Cohn et al. (1971) Master test	6/11 (55 %)	5/22 (23 %)	7/44 (16 %)
McConahay et al. (1971) Master test	17/19 (89 %)	6/12 (50 %)	19/34 (56 %)
Kassebaum et al. (1968) Near-maximal test	7/9 (78 %)	9/14 (64 %)	2/13 (16 %)
TOTAL	39/52 (75 %)	26/61 (43 %)	29/118 (25 %)

  * Luminal narrowing $\geqslant$ 50 % (Master et al., 1967; Kassebaum et al., 1968 ; McConahay et al., 1971), or $\geqslant$ 75 % (Cohn et al., 1971)

** No ST segment depression $\geqslant$ 1 mm.

In recent years, several studies have pointed out a previously unsuspected high frequency of akinetic or diskinetic ventricular zones in coronary heart disease. Dwyer (1970) has also indicated that acute myocardial ischemia caused by atrial pacing was sometimes attended by the appearance of akinetic or dyskinetic ventricular zones. The influence of chronic or reversible left ventricular akinesia or diskinesia on the exercise electrocardiogram is not yet known ; it may be speculated that these abnormalities would tend to decrease or even to suppress the ST segment depression attending exercise in coronary heart disease.

4. False positive responses.

False positive responses in the absence of any other clinical findings capable of explaining the electrocardiographic abnormality with exercise (see the paragraph « Miscellaneous conditions » below) occurred in 8 % (7/83) of the subjects presented in table 5; such false positive ST segment depression with exercise is more frequent when clinical history is negative (table 6).

The basic question is whether or not these ST segment depressions reflect myocardial ischemia. Many reports on patients with angina pectoris but no anatomical evidence of coronary disease have been published, but in a famous editorial, James (1970) stated that « the most frequent explanation for angina without coronary disease is an incorrect interpretation of the coronary arteriogram ». If this explanation is accepted then the specificity of exercise electrocardiogram is probably greater than usually thought. Another possibility is the presence of disease of the small coronary vessels, not properly visualized by coronary arteriography : this pathologic condition should be considered essentially in young patients with associated neuromuscular disease, enlarged heart, arrhythmias or conduction troubles and inverted T waves on the resting electrocardiogram (James, 1967). Finally, abnormality of the hemoglobin-oxygen dissociation curve has been reported by Eliot and Bratt (1969) as a frequent finding in women with chest pain and normal arteriography. Abnormal myocardial enzymatic activity has also been suggested in such cases (Normand et al., 1971).

B. Latent coronary heart disease.

The prevalence of ischemic ST segment depression $\geqslant$ 1 mm during or after maximal exercise tests in middle-aged clinically normal men (with a normal resting electrocardiogram) is between 5 and 13 % - table 8 (Doan et al., 1965 ; Lester et al., 1967 ; Aronow et al., 1971a). These electrocardiographic responses are often eminently transient, lasting for

TABLE 8

Incidence of ST segment depression $\geqslant$ 1 mm with exercise testing in middle-aged healthy subjects.

Source	Age years	Sex	Ischemic ST depression $\geqslant$ 1 mm	
			Submaximal tests	« Maximal » tests
Doan et al. (1965)	35-82	Male	2/201 (1 %)	18/201 (13 %)
Lester et al. (1967)	40-75	Male	1/114 (1 %)	6/114 (5 %)
Aronow et al. (1971a)	38-64	Male	4/100 (4 %)	13/100 (13 %)
TOTAL	35-82	Male	7/415 (1.7 %)	37/415 (9.1 %)
Profant et al. (1971)	30-70	Female	—	24/136* (17.6 %)

* Mean voltage of ST_B (50-69 milliseconds after nadir of S wave) of the first 100 beats after maximal exercise.

less than 30 seconds after the exercise is interrupted (Lester et al., 1967); such responses are usually much more frequent with maximal exercise testing than with submaximal exercise tests (table 8) and they are clearly age-related (fig. 8).

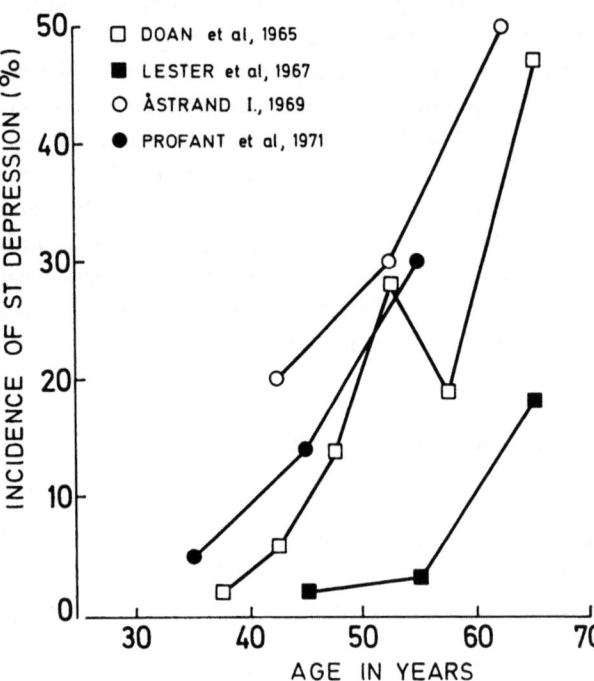

Fig. 8. — Influence of age on the incidence of ischemic electrocardiographic responses to near-maximal or maximal exercise in males (Doan et al., 1965 ; Lester et al., 1967) and females (Åstrand. 1969 ; Profant et al.. 1971).

In view of the poor prognostic significance of ichemic ST segment depression after exercise in epidemiological studies, the occurrence of an ST depression after exercise in healthy persons is now interpreted as reflecting latent coronary heart disease, but there are no anatomical studies to corroborate this interpretation. Surprisingly, the incidence of abnormal electrocardiographic responses to exercise in normal subjects is greater, in each age group, in females than in males (fig. 8); this finding is still unexplained since the incidence of overt coronary heart disease is lower for females than for males (Lepeschkin and Surawic, 1958 ; Mason et al., 1967 ; Åstrand, 1969 ; Profant et al., 1971).

C. Miscellaneous conditions.

1. Rheumatic heart disease.

Patients with rheumatic heart disease may present an ischemic electrocardiographic response to exercise. The double Master's two-step test induced an ST segment depression $\geqslant$ 1 mm in 7 out of 50 (14 %) patients with rheumatic disease and not taking digitalis ; 22 % (11/50) had an ST depression $\geqslant$ 0.5 mm (Hellerstein et al., 1961). Datey and Misra (1968) have also reported postexertional ST depression $\geqslant$ 0.5 mm in 45 % of patients with rheumatic heart disease : the mean age of these patients was 23 years and digitalis did not influence the electrocardiographic response to exercise. Unfortunately these studies did not include coronary arteriographic data. The pathophysiology of these electrocardiographic changes in patients with rheumatic heart disease is not well understood ; a possible explanation is that increased left ventricular work and poor adaptation of cardiac output to exercise cause functional myocardial ischemia in presence of a normal coronary circulation. Due to the rarity of coronary heart disease among young subjects, this mechanism is likely to explain ST depression with exercise in young patients with rheumatic heart disease ; in middle-aged patients, however, associated coronary heart disease should be eliminated by performing coronary arteriography.

2. Hypertension.

Hypertension is an important risk factor for the development of coronary heart disease (Keys, 1970a) and is associated with a higher incidence of positive electrocardiographic responses to exercise (Bellet and Roman, 1967 ; Chiang et al., 1969 ; Wong et al., 1969). Among 1346 Chinese men performing a maximal exercise test (Chiang et al., 1969), 94 (7 %) exhibited an ST depression $\geqslant$ 1 mm after maximal exercise ; the percentage of such responses was much higher (19 %) in the 119 sujects with resting hypertension (WHO criteria)*. The true significance of these abnormal electrocardiographic responses to exercise among hypertensive subjects is not easy to determine. It may be thought that these responses reflect latent coronary heart disease, often associated with hypertension ; while this explanation seems plausible for American or European populations, it is not likely in Chinese men where the incidence of coronary heart disease is low.

(*) Resting systolic pressure $\geqslant$ 160 mm Hg or diastolic pressure $\geqslant$ 95 mm Hg, or both.

An alternative explanation is to assume that ischemic ST responses with exercise mainly reflect functional myocardial ischemia due to greater systolic pressure developed and left ventricular hypertrophy; in Chinese subjects, the level of maximal systolic blood pressure, measured just after the end of exercise, is also related to the incidence of ischemic ST segment depression (Chiang et al., 1969). Wong et al. (1969) reported that uncomplicated resting hypertension in an American population (WHO criteria) did not by itself increase the incidence of electrocardiographic abnormal responses to exercise but the latter was sharply increased when electrocardiographic or radiologic signs of left ventricular hypertrophy were associated. In the study by Chiang et al. (1969) the incidence of positive responders to exercise among hypertensive subjects was also greatly increased (34 %) when resting electrocardiogram was abnormal. The interpretation of ischemic ST changes with exercise in hypertensive patients having abnormal resting electrocardiogram (the so called pattern of left ventricular strain or systolic overload) is difficult since it is not known whether the ischemic changes with exercise represent simply an accentuation of the left ventricular strain (which is a secondary trouble of repolarisation) or if they indicate the occurrence of myocardial ischemia (primary trouble of repolarization). It seems prudent to conclude that the interpretation of electrocardiographic responses to exercise in hypertensive disease is still empirical; the need for studies correlating hemodynamic data, coronary arteriographic findings and electrocardiographic responses to exercise is obvious.

3. Congenital abnormalities of the coronary arteries.

Congenital abnormalities of the coronary arteries should be considered a possible cause of ischemic electrocardiographic response to exercise among young subjects. Among 35 patients with angina pectoris (mean age = 43 years ; 40 % women), 9 (25 %)

had congenital abnormalities of the coronary arteries capable of explaining their complaints (Hillestad and Eie, 1970).

4. «Non specific» electrocardiographic abnormalities.

« Non specific » electrocardiographic abnormalities are commonly encountered at rest in young patients, often women, with atypical complaints, normal heart volume and sometimes clinical signs of increased sympathetic tone (Freteur et al., 1966 ; Furberg, 1968); these abnormalities mostly concern the T waves which are inverted, but the ST segment is also sometimes involved. Such abnormalities are often exaggerated in upright posture. Several tests are used to differentiate these non specific ECG changes from those of organic origin : uncharacteristic ST - T abnormalities are often corrected in the fasting condition, with exercise, after ingestion of potassium or administration of a beta blocking agent. Freteur et al. (1970) reported normalization of the electrocardiogram after a multistage test of maximal exercise in 90 % (19/21) of their subjects while all tracings became normal when such exercise was performed after ingestion of potassium ; the specificity of maximal exercise test after potassium has still to be established, however, since the tracings of some angina patients are also corrected with potassium (Solvay and Denolin, 1967 ; Goenen et al., 1970). Furberg (1967) reported correction of all aspecific ECG changes by exercise during beta-adrenergic blockade (10 to 20 mg of propranolol one hour before the test); in a group of coronary patients beta-adrenergic blockade never abolished ST segment depression during or immediately after the exercise test. Furberg's data (1967 ; 1968) in angina patients conflict, however, with many other studies which have clearly indicated that beta-blocking agents often improved or even normalized the exercise electrocardiogram of coronary patients (see the next paragraph).

INFLUENCE OF THERAPEUTICS ON EXERTIONAL ELECTROCARDIOGRAM

Exertional and postexertional ST segment depression can be modified by several therapeutics such as the administration of drugs, physical training or surgical myocardial revascularization.

A. Nitroglycerin.

Nitroglycerin diminishes the importance of the ST

segment depression caused by submaximal exercise in coronary patients (Kinsella et al., 1962 ; McAlpin et al., 1965); it also decreases the importance of the ST segment depression attending maximal exercise and increases the symptom-limited capacity of angina patients (Detry and Bruce, 1971a). These effects of nitroglycerin on the magnitude of exertional ST segment depression do not result from lower heart rate or pressure-rate product at submaximal or maximal exercise (table 9), because lower depression of the ST segment with nitroglycerin occurs despite unchanged or even greater values of the pressure-rate product and the relationship between the magnitude of the ST segment depression during exercise and the pressure-rate product (fig. 9) is consequently modified (Detry and Bruce, 1971a).

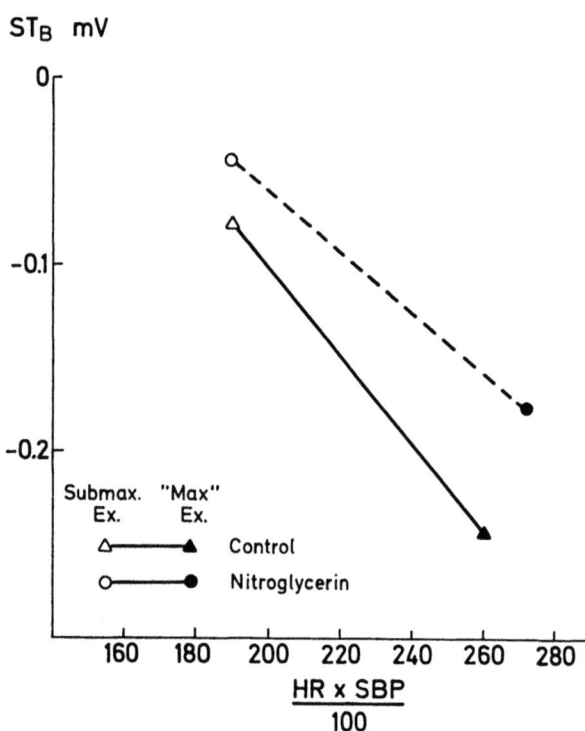

Fig. 9. — Effects of sublingual nitroglycerin on the relationship between the magnitude of the exertional ST segment depression and the pressure-rate product (heart rate x systolic blood pressure/100) in 37 coronary patients ; submaximal exercise refers to the last minute of the first stage of the Bruce's multistage treadmill test. The electrocardiograms were analyzed by a computer averaging technic. Absolute values and statistics are presented in table 9 where ST_B is also defined (from Detry and Bruce, 1971a).

Since nitroglycerin does not appear to produce a significant increase in the coronary blood flow of patients with coronary heart disease (Gorlin et al., 1959 ; Rowe et al., 1961 ; Bing et al., 1964 ; Bernstein et al., 1966; Parker et al., 1971) an alternative explanation is that this drug decreases the myocardial oxygen requirements despite unchanged or even greater pressure-rate product by decreasing ventricular volume. At rest nitroglycerin decreases heart volume (Williams et al., 1965 ; Frick et al., 1968 ; Goldstein

et al., 1971a) and this action has been attributed to peripheral venous pooling of blood secondary to increased venous compliance (Wilkins et al., 1937 ; Åblad, 1963 ; Mason and Braunwald, 1965) ; similar effects of nitroglycerin on heart volume (Goldstein et al., 1971a) and venous compliance (Detry et al., 1972b) have also been observed during exercise. Decreased heart volume during exercise with nitroglycerin certainly contributes to the lessening of the depression of the ST segment ; other mechanisms such as a modification of the distribution of the coronary blood flow, could also play a role (Becker et al., 1971 ; Winbury et al., 1971). From a practical point of view, the action of nitroglycerin on exercise electrocardiogram indicates that in coronary patients the diagnostic sensitivity of exercise testing will be decreased if the test is performed less than 1 to 2 hours after absorption of this drug.

B. Beta blocking agents.

Propranolol increases the exercise capacity of angina patients and decreases the importance of the exertional ST segment depression. Heart rate and pressure-rate product at the onset of angina pectoris are significantly decreased by propranolol (Russek, 1968 ; Battock et al., 1969 ; Gianelly et al., 1969). For instance in 26 angina patients, maximal heart rate was 32 beats lower (108 versus 140) one hour after oral administration of 40 to 80 mg of propranolol ; in addition, anginal pain was prevented in 8 of these patients (Russek, 1968). At the same time the amount of ST segment depression at the maximal exercise level (anginal threshold) is significantly decreased after propranolol (Russek, 1968 ; Gianelly et al., 1969 ; Battock et al., 1969 ; Lichtlen et al., 1971). It is still unclear whether or not the relationship of the heart rate or pressure-rate product to the importance of exertional ST segment depression is modified with propranolol, although data presented by Battock et al. (1969) suggest this.

Practolol is a beta blocking agent which has a selective action on cardiac beta-adrenergic receptors and no quinidine-like action ; it also differs from propranolol by its much longer half-life (Dunlop and Shanks, 1968 ; Fitzgerald and Scales, 1968). The action of practolol on the exercise tolerance of angina pectoris is similar to that of propranolol : the maximal heart rate and the maximal ST segment depression are indeed lower after practolol while the exercise capacity is increased (Areskog and Adolfsson, 1969 ; Frick and Kattila, 1970 ; Sowton et al., 1971). Rousseau et al., (1972a) made a detailed examina-

TABLE 9

Effects of sublingual nitroglycerin (0.4 mg) on the pressure-rate product and the importance of the ST segment depression during submaximal and maximal exercise (from Detry and Bruce, 1971a).

		$\dfrac{HR \times SBP}{100}$	ST_B mV ***
Healed myocardial infarction (n = 18)			
Submaximal* :	Control	183	— 0.035
	Nitroglycerin	187	— 0.012
	P **	NS	NS
Maximal :	Control	281	— 0.254
	Nitroglycerin	279	— 0.166
	P	NS	< 0.005
Angina pectoris (n = 19)			
Submaximal :	Control	198	— 0.120
	Nitroglycerin	193	— 0.072
	P	NS	< 0.0005
Maximal :	Control	243	— 0.234
	Nitroglycerin	266	— 0.188
	P	< 0.001	< 0.0005
All patients (n = 37)			
Submaximal :	Control	191	— 0.079
	Nitroglycerin	190	— 0.043
	P	NS	< 0.005
Maximal :	Control	261	— 0.244
	Nitroglycerin	272	—0,177
	P	NS	< 0.0001

* Last minute of the first stage of the multistage treadmill test of Bruce (table 3).

** Paired *T* test.

*** ST_B refers to the mean voltage of the ST segment from 50 to 69 msec after the nadir of S wave, with the P-R interval as zero reference voltage.

tion of the effects of practolol on the ST segment depression attending submaximal exercise : the pressure-time index (heart rate x systolic aortic pressure x ejection time) and the importance of the ST segment depression were both significantly ($P<0.001$) decreased with practolol. Practolol also modified the relationship between the pressure-time index and the magnitude of ST segment depression during exercise : at a given level of pressure-time index, the ST segment was always less depressed after practolol (Rousseau et al., 1972a).

The mechanisms of action of beta blocking agents on the exertional ST segment depression in coronary patients remain unclear. This problem is largely due to the fact that beta blocking drugs have opposite effects on two important determinants of the myocardial oxygen requirements which are not taken into account in the pressure-rate product : heart volume tends indeed to increase after beta blockade while myocardial contractility is decreased (Chamberlain, 1966 ; Graham et al., 1967). In any event, from an electrocardiographic point of view, one is faced with an alternative. If the importance of ST segment depression remains a reliable index of myocardial ischemia, it must be concluded that, after beta blockade, angina pectoris is precipitated for unknown reasons at a lesser degree of myocardial ischemia. On the other hand if angina pectoris occurs with beta blocking agents at an unchanged degree of myocardial hypoxia, then the amount of ST segment depression during exercise is no longer a satisfactory sign of myocardial hypoxia.

The exact role of asynergy of left ventricular contraction induced by beta adrenergic blockade (Helfant et al., 1971a) on the electrocardiographic response to exercise also remains to be established. It has also been suggested that beta-blocking agents produce a redistribution of coronary blood flow to improve perfusion of the subendocardial regions (Winbury et al., 1971).

Since propranolol and practolol often suppress the ischemic electrocardiographic response to exercise in patients with documented coronary heart disease, it is essential to consider the possible role of these drugs in the interpretation of the exertional electrocardiogram.

C. Digitalis.

Digitalis causes false positive electrocardiographic responses to exercise, for such responses occurred in 12 out of 25 (48 %) normal young subjects whose control exercise electrocardiogram was otherwise normal (Kawai and Hultgren, 1964 ; Hirsch, 1965); these false positive responses also occur in the subjects whose resting ECG does not show digitalis induced ST segment depression (Kawai and Hultgren, 1964). In patients with rheumatic heart disease, however, digitalis did not influence the electrocardiographic response to exercise (Hellerstein et al., 1961 ; Datey and Misra, 1968). These effects of digitalis on the ST segment are usually attributed to intramyocardial potassium depletion, for oral administration of potassium sometimes prevents abnormal exercise responses due to digitalis ; however, this preventive action of potassium is not constant (Kawai and Hultgren, 1964). From a practical point of view, one should consider that the ST segment during or after exercise is not interpretable in patients receiving digitalis ; this drug should therefore be discontinued 2 to 4 weeks before diagnostic exercise testing, according to the type of digitalis used.

D. Physical training.

After physical training of coronary patients, the magnitude of the ST segment depression at a given submaximal level of exercise is decreased (Barry et al.. 1966 ; Hellerstein et al., 1967 ; Gottheiner, 1968 ;

Salzman et al., 1969) but the pressure-rate product, tension-time index and presumably myocardial oxygen requirements are also decreased (Frick and Katila, 1968 ; Clausen et al., 1969 ; Detry et al., 1971 ; Rousseau et al., 1972b). At the level of maximal exercise however, the ST segment was more depressed after physical training in 14 patients and the relationship between the importance of the ST segment depression during exercise and the pressure-rate product was unchanged - table 10, fig. 10 (Detry and Bruce, 1971b). Modification of the electrocardiographic responses to exercise after physical training consequently appears to result mostly from changes in heart rate and blood pressure responses to exercise rather than from an improved coronary circulation ; in other words the changes in the electrocardiographic response to submaximal exercise cannot be interpreted as indicating the development of a collateral coronary circulation after physical training.

TABLE 10

Effects of physical training on the pressure-rate product and the importance of the ST segment depression during submaximal and maximal exercise in 14 patients with coronary heart disease (from Detry and Bruce, 1971b).

	$\dfrac{HR \times SBP}{100}$	ST_B mV***
Submaximal *		
Before training	179	— 0.095
After training	155	— 0.027
P **	< 0.02	< 0.05
Maximal :		
Before training	226	— 0.202
After training	241	— 0.262
P	< 0.02	< 0.005

* Last minute of the first stage of the multistage treadmill test of Bruce (table 3).

** Paired T test.

*** ST_B refers to the mean voltage of the ST segment from 50 to 69 msec after the nadir of S wave, with the P-R interval as zero reference voltage.

The effects of physical training on the exercise electrocardiogram consequently differ greatly from those of nitroglycerin ; the actions of these two therapeutics on the exercise electrocardiogram have been

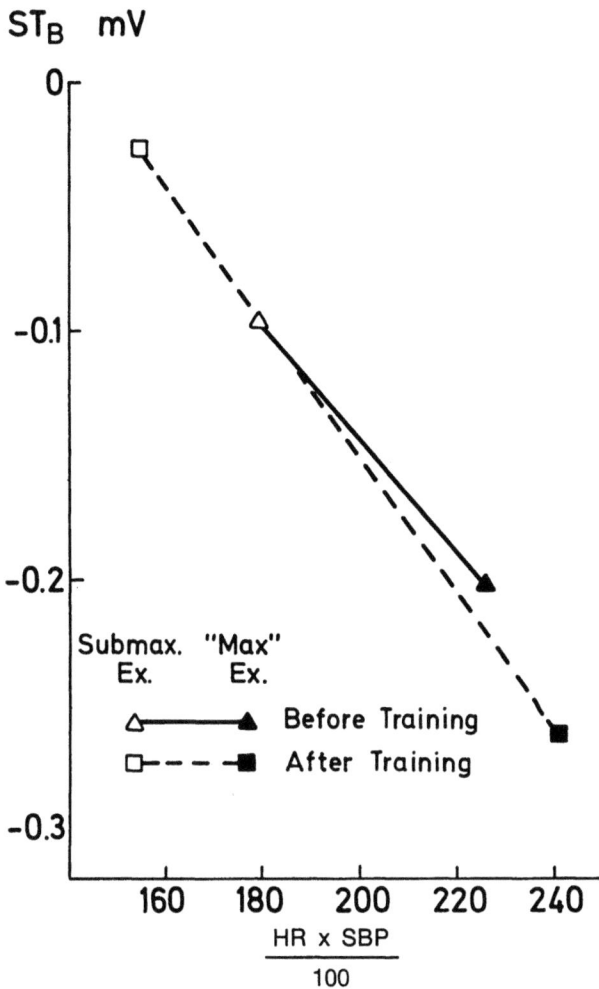

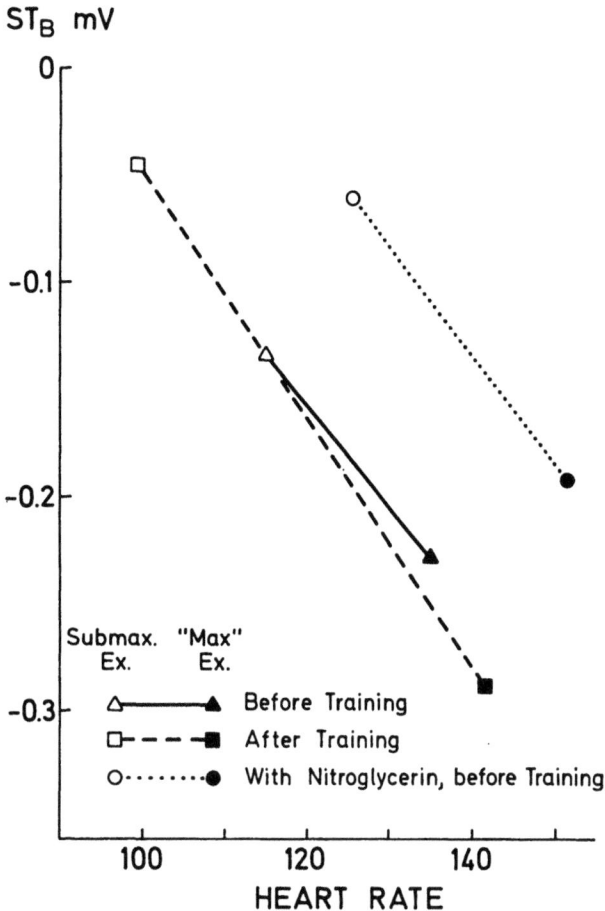

Fig. 10. — Effects of a 3 months physical training program on the relationship between the magnitude of exertional ST segment depression and the pressure-rate product in 14 coronary patients (see legend of fig. 9). Absolute values and statistics are presented in table 10 (from Detry and Bruce, 1971b).

Fig. 11. — Effects of nitroglycerin and physical training on heart rate and ST segment depression during exercise in 9 subjects, 7 of whom had angina pectoris. Submaximal exercise refers to the last minute of the first stage of the multistage treadmill test of Bruce. All heart rate or ST segment data collected after training or with nitroglycerin were significantly different from those collected before training at the 0.05 significance level, except for the ST segment depression at the maximal exercise level with nitroglycerin (from Detry and Bruce, 1971c).

compared in a small group of 9 patients (fig. 11) and the result of this comparison confirms the data previously collected in 2 separate larger groups of different patients (Detry and Bruce, 1971c).

E. Surgical myocardial « revascularisation ».

Little information is yet available on the effects of surgical treatment of coronary insufficiency on the exercise electrocardiogram. Among 34 patients treated by internal mammary artery implantation who had pre - and postoperative angiographic studies, 29 had

a persistent positive response to exercise after surgery : in 24 of these 29 patients (83 %) the implants were occluded or no angiographic evidence of revascularization was present (Kassebaum et al., 1969). Five subjects presented a reversal of their electrocardiographic response to exercise from positive before the operation to negative postoperatively : in all these patients development of collaterals was demonstrated angiographically. Bloomer et al., (1970) reported that electrocardiographic response to exercise was improved after arterial myocardial implants in 36 of 51 patients with patent implant ; however, in 7 of these

36 patients (19 %) no effective myocardial perfusion through the implant could be demonstrated. On the other hand, the exercise electrocardiogram was not improved in 15 patients despite the fact that 13 (86 %) demonstrated improved myocardial perfusion after surgery.

Discrepancies between the few published studies and the small number of cases reported preclude an accurate estimation of the sensitivity and specificity of exercise electrocardiography in the assessment of postoperative results. Furthermore, no data are yet available with saphenous venous grafting which appears a much more promising surgical approach than revascularization with arterial implants.

CHAPTER III

Physical work capacity in coronary heart disease

The most important objective for exercise testing of patients with documented coronary heart disease is the measurement of their physical work capacity. In healthy subjects, the most accurate expression of the physical work capacity is undoubtedly the maximal oxygen intake ($V_{O2,max}$), also designated the maximal aerobic power, the maximal aerobic work capacity or the functional aerobic power. The maximal oxygen intake is a physiological parameter and this term can be used only when several conditions are fulfilled ; as will be discussed later, the oxygen intake measured at the maximal exercise level in cardiac patients does not always satisfy the criteria and in these conditions the term of symptom limited oxygen consumption ($V_{O2,SL}$) is preferable. To avoid confusion we will use the term of physical capacity in a wide sense to express the functional capacity of a subject normal or sick ; the term $V_{O2,max}$ will be used only when the physiological requirements are satisfied.

The purposes of determining the physical work capacity of coronary patients can be summarized as follows. It is the only way to estimate accurately the functional impairment due to the disease ; the clinical findings at rest and the history of the patient provide only an approximation of the functional capacity of a patient, and direct measurement is required to prevent overestimation and, perhaps more important for the rehabilitation of patients, to prevent underestimation. With serial measurements it is also possible to observe changes which may be attributed to the natural history of the disease or to the effects of a therapy. Finally, quantitative assessment of physical work capacity is the best way to determine the capacity of an individual to perform a given task.

The estimation of the functional impairment of cardiac patients is possible only by comparison with data collected in healthy control subjects. The first section of this chapter will therefore be devoted to the physical capacity of normal subjects, which will be used as a reference frame ; the methods for determining the physical capacity of cardiac patients and normal subjects(*) do not differ substantially and they will be considered in this first section. The second section will cover the physical work capacity of coronary patients.

PHYSICAL WORK CAPACITY OF HEALTHY SUBJECTS

The maximal oxygen intake is the most reliable index for physical fitness. It is based on the classical observation by Lijestrand and Stenström (1920) and Hill et al. (1924) that with increasing work load, the oxygen consumption reaches a plateau which represents the maximal aerobic capacity for an individual. By definition, the $V_{O2,max}$ is « *the highest oxygen uptake the individual can attain during physical work breathing air at sea level* » (Åstrand and Rodahl, 1970). An objective criterion is needed to determine whether or not the $V_{O2,max}$ has in fact been measured : this is the demonstration of a levelling off or even a decrease of the O_2 consumption despite a further increase in the workload. Since this O_2 consumption plateau is not always clearly demonstrated, another helpful criterion is the level of blood lactate during early recovery : when it reaches 90 to 100 mg/100 ml blood after exercise performed with large muscle groups in young subjects, the workload has usually been of sufficient intensity

---

(*) A good part of the methodological problems have already been considered in chapter 2 and will therefore not be further discussed.

to elicit $\dot{V}_{O2,max}$ (Åstrand, 1952). In older subjects lactate levels of 70 to 80 mg/100 ml blood often attend a demonstrated levelling off of the oxygen consumption (Åstrand, 1960). Subsidiary criteria are a respiratory quotient higher than 1.15 and a pulse rate in excess of the predicted maximal values. The workload which completely exhausts a subject within 5 to 6 minutes is usually eliciting the $\dot{V}_{O2,max}$ but this criterion is subjective and relies upon full cooperation from the subject.

The methods used to measure $\dot{V}_{O2,max}$ directly or to predict it will be briefly reviewed and the physiological implications of $\dot{V}_{O2,max}$ will then be discussed.

A. Methods.

The only way to determine the $\dot{V}_{O2,max}$ of an individual is to measure it directly, which requires testing up to the maximal exercise level. Classical methods use several workloads separated by a long rest period, while with uninterrupted tests the $\dot{V}_{O2,max}$ can be measured in a single session. Indirect estimations of the $\dot{V}_{O2,max}$ from submaximal exercise data are also used but these methods have inherent limitations.

1. Direct measurement of maximal oxygen intake.

Classically, the measurement of the $\dot{V}_{O2,max}$ requires the demonstration of a levelling off of the oxygen consumption and thus testing at 2 or more separated near-maximal, maximal or supra-maximal workloads ; these high intensity exercises should always be preceded by a warming up exercise of submaximal intensity, and they have to be performed on separate days (Åstrand, 1952 ; Taylor et al., 1955). To elicit maximal oxygen intake, a large percentage of the total muscle mass should be used ; $\dot{V}_{O2,max}$ during arm exercise is lower than during leg exercise but addition of arm work to leg work does not increase the $\dot{V}_{O2,max}$ significantly (Åstrand and Saltin, 1961b). Taylor et al. (1955) use a treadmill with fixed speed at 7 m.p.h. and increase the grade of the treadmill by steps of 2.5 % ; each step lasts 2.45 min and they consider that an O_2 consumption plateau has been reached when the difference in O_2 consumption between 2 separate exercise levels does not exceed 150 ml/min or 2.1 ml/kg. Åstrand P.O. (1952) and Åstrand I. (1960) use the bicycle ergometer and separated workloads of progressive intensity (steps of 25 to 50 watts for 6 minutes) until a plateau in oxygen consumption is demonstrated. The duration of the workload is not critical since maximal oxygen intake can be elicited by very heavy exercise main-

tained for 3 minutes, or less heavy exercise for up to 8 minutes (Åstrand and Saltin, 1961a) ; the absolute intensity of the workload causing the $\dot{V}_{O2,max}$ will therefore vary with the duration of the exercise test.

The demonstration of a levelling off of the oxygen intake is a time consuming procedure both for the researcher and the subject, since the heavy exercise tests should ideally be performed on separate days. Accordingly efforts have been made to develop uninterrupted multistage tests to measure the $\dot{V}_{O2,max}$ in a single session.

In uninterrupted tests, the intensity of the exercise is increased in a stepwise fashion without any intervening rest periods and the subject is asked to push himself up to his maximal limits : the end point of the test will therefore be determined by the subject himself and his motivation is consequently essential. Both the treadmill and the bicycle ergometer can be used to measure the $\dot{V}_{O2,max}$ in continuous tests of progressive severity (Shephard et al., 1968). The $\dot{V}_{O2,max}$ measured with continuous tests does not differ from that determined with the classical methods (Shepard et al., 1968 ; Bruce, 1970); Pirnay et al. (1966) even reported that uninterrupted tests of maximal exercise elicited a higher $\dot{V}_{O2,max}$ (+ 6.4 %; $P < 0.02$) due to higher maximal heart rate (+ 4.6 beats/min ; $P < 0.02$). Several types of uninterrupted tests have been described ; in the multisage test of Bruce, the grade and the speed of the treadmill are increased every 3 minutes (table 3) while Pirnay et al. (1966) maintain a constant grade of 10 % and increase the speed by 2 km/hour every 2 minutes. Bruce (1971) recently published nomograms to estimate the physical work capacity from the duration of the multistage treadmill test, taking account of the age, sex and physical activity status. The rate at which the workload is increased does not appear critical for the measurement of the $\dot{V}_{O2,max}$ although the maximal heart rate is higher when the total duration of the test increases (Bottin et al., 1970).

At the end of uninterrupted maximal exercise tests, the O_2 consumption often tends to level off despite continuous increase of the external workload and a plateau of O_2 consumption can therefore be demonstrated (Pirnay et al., 1966 ; Bruce, 1970); when the bicycle ergometer is used, one should always check that the levelling off of the O_2 consumption does not in fact correspond to a slow decrease in the rate of pedalling.

The *type of ergometer* used to measure the $\dot{V}_{O2,max}$ is important since, with both discontinuous and continuous procedures, the treadmill gives higher values than the bicycle ergometer (Åstrand and Saltin, 1961b ; Shephard et al., 1968 ; Hermansen and Saltin, 1969) ; the values obtained with stepping lie between those collected with bicycling and running uphill (Shephard et al., 1968). It is not clear why $\dot{V}_{O2,max}$ measured with a treadmill are higher than when a bicycle ergometer is used ; in 13 young normal subjects the difference ($+ 6\%$; $P < 0.001$) was due to slightly higher maximal heart rate ($+ 1.5\%$; NS) and mostly to greater stroke volume ($+ 4.5\%$; $P < 0.005$) on the treadmill (Hermansen et al., 1970). The difference between treadmill and bicycle ergometer $\dot{V}_{O2,max}$ is not large but it does preclude the interchangeable use of both methods in longitudinal studies. The posture is of greater importance since $\dot{V}_{O2,max}$ is significantly lower ($- 15\%$) during supine cycling as compared with upright exercise ; this difference is attended by a lower maximal heart rate during supine exercise (Åstrand and Saltin, 1961b).

2. Prediction of maximal oxygen intake.

In 1954 Åstrand and Ryhming proposed a nomogram for calculation of the $\dot{V}_{O2,max}$ from the heart rate and the oxygen consumption or the workload during a submaximal exercise test ; this nomogram assumes a linear relationship between the $\dot{V}_{O2}$ and the heart rate from submaximal up to maximal exercise levels and a small variation of the maximal heart rate around the mean value of 195 in the 18 - 30 age group. In 1960, Åstrand adjusted the nomogram and introduced a factor designed to correct for the influence of age so that it can be used in all age groups ; she also stressed that only submaximal heart rates higher than 125 beats/min should be used for the prediction of the $\dot{V}_{O2,max}$. Åstrand (1960) pointed out that under carefully standardized experimental conditions, the standard deviation of the predicted $\dot{V}_{O2,max}$ was important, varying from ± 10 to $\pm 15\%$, and stated clearly that this method allowed only a rough prediction of $\dot{V}_{O2,max}$; this considerable error in the prediction of the $\dot{V}_{O2,max}$ results mostly from the wide standard deviation of the mean maximal heart rate. Rowell et al. (1964c) compared the measured $\dot{V}_{O2,max}$ to that predicted from the Åstrand-Ryhming nomogram or that obtained by extrapolation up to the measured maximal heart rate of the slope relating heart rate and O_2 consumption during submaximal exercise ; predicted and extrapolated $\dot{V}_{O2,max}$ underestimated the true $\dot{V}_{O2,max}$ by 26.8 % and 23.3 % in untrained subjects.

Underestimation was less after physical conditioning but still above 13 %.

The heart rate response to submaximal exercise is influenced by several factors, such as dehydration, exposure to a hot environment, prolongation or repetition of exercise or non-specific stresses such as anxiety due to a lack of familiarization with the testing procedure. All these factors do not modify the actual $\dot{V}_{O2,max}$ significantly but they considerably change the value of the $\dot{V}_{O2,max}$ as predicted from the Åstrand-Ryhming nomogram; it should be stressed, however, that dehydration and exposure to hot environment, although not affecting the $\dot{V}_{O2,max}$, significantly decrease the capacity to perform prolonged work (Rowell, 1962 ; Rowell et al., 1964c ; Saltin 1964a, 1964b ; Saltin and Stenberg, 1964 ; Pirnay et al., 1970a).

Several authors have proposed estimating the physical work capacity from the oxygen consumption or the workload corresponding to a heart rate of 170 (Sjöstrand, 1947; Wahlund, 1948 ; Messin et al., 1965) ; this physical work capacity at a heart rate of 170 (PWC_{170}) is either directly measured or extrapolated from exercise tests of lower intensity. The value of 170 beats/min has been chosen since it should represent the limit above which prolonged exercise is not tolerated. All the limitations for the prediction of the $\dot{V}_{O2,max}$ with the Åstrand-Ryhming nomogram also apply to the estimation of the PWC_{170} ; furthermore the PWC_{170} does not take into account the physiological decrease in maximal heart rate with age so that physical capacity of young subjects is often underestimated while that of older subjects can be overestimated (Pirnay et al., 1970b).

B. Physiological implications of maximal oxygen intake.

According to the Fick principle, the $\dot{V}_{O2,max}$ is equal to the product of the maximal cardiac output and the maximal $a\text{-}\bar{v}_{O2}$ difference. The $\dot{V}_{O2,max}$ is therefore limited by the interplay of several factors, such as the maximal heart rate, the stroke volume at the maximal exercise level and the maximal $a\text{-}\bar{v}_{O2}$ difference ; the latter depends on the hemoglobin content of the blood, the redistribution of cardiac output away from non-working beds and the extraction of oxygen by the working muscles. Under normal conditions, the $\dot{V}_{O2,max}$ is not limited by pulmonary factors (Mitchell et al., 1958 ; Saltin, 1964b).

Which factor is the most important in the determination of the $\dot{V}_{O2,max}$ is still disputed. Quantitatively the contribution of the increase in cardiac output from resting upright condition up to the maximal exercise level is usually greater than that of the widening of the a-$\bar{v}_{O_2}$ difference; comparison of resting and maximal exercise data reveals that at the $\dot{V}_{O_2,max}$ level, the cardiac output is 4.5 times greater than at rest, while the a-$\bar{v}_{O_2}$ difference is only 2.4 times wider (Mitchell et al., 1958; Rowell, 1969). Accordingly, several authors consider that $\dot{V}_{O_2,max}$ is mostly a measure of the functional capacity of the cardiovascular system, and in this conception the maximal pumping capacity of the heart would be the factor limiting maximal performance (Taylor et al., 1955; Saltin, 1964b; Shephard et al., 1968; Rowell, 1969; Grimby and Saltin, 1971). An alternative hypothesis is that $\dot{V}_{O_2,max}$ is not limited by the maximal oxygen transport but rather by the maximal metabolic rate of the working muscles; this opinion is supported by the fact that wide variations in arterial O_2 content, and thus in the amount of O_2 transported by the circulation, did not cause significant changes in the aerobic work capacity (Kaijser, 1970; Pirnay et al., 1972). The effects of physical training on the maximal a-$\bar{v}_{O_2}$ difference and on the enzymatic respiratory system of the muscle also support this hypothesis (see chapter 4). These two working hypotheses on the factors limiting maximal aerobic performances are not contradictory, however, and until clear experimental exidence demonstrates that $\dot{V}_{O_2,max}$ is limited by a single factor it is most logical to consider that the maximal aerobic capacity depends on both central and peripheral factors.

As pointed out in chapter I, the relative severity of an exercise determines several hemodynamic adjustments: the redistribution of cardiac output away from splanchnic and renal regions is indeed related to the percentage of $\dot{V}_{O_2,max}$. The fraction of the total cardiac output available for the working muscles is therefore determined by the relative intensity of the exercise (Rowell, 1969); the total a-$\bar{v}_{O_2}$ difference is also linearly related to the percent of $\dot{V}_{O_2,max}$ (Åstrand et al., 1964). When subjects with very low $\dot{V}_{O_2,max}$, such as patients with mitral stenosis, are compared with sedentary normals or athletes, it is seen that their overall circulatory adaptation to exercise is similar when workloads of the same relative intensity are compared (Blackmon et al., 1967; Rowell, 1969). It follows that, to compare subjects with different degrees of physical fitness, the $\dot{V}_{O_2,max}$ should be taken into account and exercise of the same relative intensity should be used.

1. Influence of age, sex and weight.

The $\dot{V}_{O_2,max}$ decreases with age and is constantly higher in males than in females (Åstrand, 1952). The hemodynamic determinants of $\dot{V}_{O_2,max}$ in sedentary subjects of different ages and sexes are presented in table 11. The decrease in $\dot{V}_{O_2,max}$ with age is caused mostly by a decrease in the maximal heart rate with age (fig. 4); this phenomeon is present in both sexes and is of the same magnitude in untrained and well-trained subjects (Grimby et al., 1966; Ekblom and Hermansen, 1968; Lester et al., 1968). Stroke volume also tends to be lower in older subjects, while a-$\bar{v}_{O_2}$ difference at maximal exercise does not appear to be altered by aging; the exact evolution of stroke volume and maximal a-$\bar{v}_{O_2}$ difference with age should, however, be further defined by longitudinal studies.

In all age groups, women have lower $\dot{V}_{O_2,max}$ than men, even when correction is made for the difference in body weight; the lower $\dot{V}_{O_2,max}$ of women results from their lower maximal a-$\bar{v}_{O_2}$ difference related to their lower hemoglobin content,

TABLE 11

Hemodynamic determinants of $\dot{V}_{O_2,max}$ in sedentary healthy subjects.

Source	Number of subjects	Sex	Age years	$\dot{V}_{O_2,max}$ l/min	HR beats/min	Qs ml/beat	Q l/min	a-$\bar{v}_{O_2}$ diff. ml/100 ml
Saltin (1969) *	17	M	21.6	3.11	196	110	21.5	14.4
Hartley et al. (1969)	13	M	47	2.68	182	103	18.7	14.4
Kiblom and Astrand (1971)	9	F	33	1.94	184	78	14.3	13.6
Kiblom and Astrand (1971)	4	F	55	1.58	167	69	11.5	13.8

* Average values of data collected by Rowell (1962), Ekblom et al. (1968) and Saltin et al. (1968).
Abbreviations: HR = Heart Rate; Qs = Stroke Volume; Q = Cardiac Output.

and also from their lower stroke volume (table 11); the latter is partly determined by the lower heart volume of females (Åstrand et al., 1964).

The $\dot{V}_{O2,max}$ is related to the body weight ($r = 0.63$) especially when it is expressed as fat free body weight ($r = 0.85$) taken as an index of the mass of working muscles ; if $\dot{V}_{O2,max}$ is used to determine the fitness of an invidual to perform tasks involving the displacement of the body, then it should be expressed in ml/kg of body weight (Åstrand, 1952; Buskirk and Taylor, 1957). Obesity by itself does not influence the $\dot{V}_{O2,max}$ since sedentary subjects with different percentages of body fat have the same $\dot{V}_{O2,max}$ when it is expressed in ml/kg of fat free body weight ; the capacity of the cardiovascular system to transport oxygen and that of the muscles to consume it is therefore not altered directly by obesity. Obese subjects are, however, limited in the accomplishment of a given task since they have to carry a load of fat which does not contribute to the $\dot{V}_{O2,max}$.

The $\dot{V}_{O2,max}$ is also greatly influenced by the degree of physical training : it decreases with inactivity or bed rest and increases with physical conditioning. These particular aspects will be developed in chapter 4.

2. Maximal oxygen intake and capacity for prolonged work.

The capacity to perform prolonged submaximal work depends on the relative intensity of the workload, i.e. on the percentage of the $\dot{V}_{O2,max}$ required, and on the degree of physical training. For a full working day of 8 hours, the mean severity of exercise that can be performed by untrained subjects without undue fatigue corresponds to approximately 35 % of the $\dot{V}_{O2,max}$ (Michael et al., 1961 ; Bonjer, 1968 ; Falls, 1969) ; Åstrand (1960) reported that work at

50 % of $\dot{V}_{O2,max}$ was well tolerated for 1 hour, but its prolongation for 8 hours caused a progressive increase in heart rate and rectal temperature and that subjective fatigue was mentioned by 3 of the 4 subjects studied. The measurement of heart rate during steady state exercise is an easy way to determine the capacity for prolonged work : according to Michael et al. (1961) a heart rate of 120 beats/min can be maintained without fatigue for 8 hours while a heart rate of 140 beats/min cannot be tolerated for more than 4 hours. Very well trained subjects are able to work for longer periods of time and at higher percentage of $\dot{V}_{O2,max}$ than unfit persons (Åstrand and Rodahl, 1970) ; the great motivation of athletes and their tolerance of discomfort probably account partly for their greater endurance.

All the above mentioned studies are based on experiments with prolonged work at a constant workload. In fact, most if not all professional tasks are essentially discontinuous, heavy work being followed by light work or by a recovery period. In estimating the severity of professional work, therefore, one has to consider the mean energy requirements since peak workloads do not usually limit normal subjects, although they do become an essential problem in patients with angina pectoris or intermittent claudication. In evaluating the severity of a given task, environmental factors (temperature, humidity), psychological tension and isometric exercise which cause all a higher cardiac cost without much influencing the oxygen cost, have also to be taken into consideration.

In any case, European society is moving towards the progressive disappearance of very heavy professional occupations ; Blomqvist (1971) considers that most American professional activities can now be classified as sedentary or light.

PHYSICAL WORK CAPACITY OF CORONARY PATIENTS

The physical work capacity of patients with coronary heart disease is lower than that of healthy subjects of similar age and sex (table 12) ; the values measured in 23 patients without angina pectoris are 80 % of the normal values predicted from age (McDonough et al., 1970) while those of 32 patients limited by angina pectoris are only 62 % of the predicted normal values (Detry and Bruce, 1971a).

The first problem is to determine whether the values presented in table 12 represent true $\dot{V}_{O2,max}$ or not. Oxygen consumption was measured during the last 3 minutes of the multistage treadmill test in 19 patients without angina pectoris and in 27 patients with exertional angina pectoris (Detry and Bruce, 1971a). The patients without angina pectoris present a clear levelling-off of the O_2 consumption during the last minute of the test (fig. 12); the

TABLE 12

Effects of coronary heart disease (CHD) on physical work capacity measured during a multistage treadmill test (from Detry and Bruce, 1971a).

	Age years	$\dot{V}_{O2,max}$ or $\dot{V}_{O2,SL}$ ml/kg . min	Maximal heart rate beats/min
Normal subjects n = 12	46.2	34.5	170
CHD without angina pectoris n = 23	50.3	28.1	165
CHD with angina pectoris n = 32	51.4	21.2	139

values measured during the forelast minute of the test are indeed 99 % of those collected during the last minute. In these conditions the $\dot{V}_{O2}$ measured during the last minute of the multistage treadmill test in patients without angina pectoris represents true $\dot{V}_{O2,max}$. On the other hand, patients limited by angina pectoris do not present a plateau of oxygen consumption at the end of the test which, by definition, was interrupted for typical chest pain (fig. 12): the $\dot{V}_{O2}$ increased continuously until the end of the exercise test and the values collected during the forelast minute are 95 % of the maximal values during the last minute of the test. The $\dot{V}_{O2}$ measured at the maximal exercise level in angina patients cannot therefore be designated $\dot{V}_{O2,max}$ but should rather be termed symptom limited maximal oxygen intake or $\dot{V}_{O2,SL}$ (Detry and Bruce, 1971b).

Since $\dot{V}_{O2,SL}$ does not have the same physiological meaning as $\dot{V}_{O2,max}$, the factors limiting the physical work capacity of coronary patients with or without angina pectoris will be discussed separately.

A. Coronary patients without angina pectoris.

Patients with healed myocardial infarction have lower $\dot{V}_{O2,max}$ than healthy control subjects (table 12); the factors responsible for the functional impairment of these patients are not yet exactly defined. Accurate analysis of these limiting factors would indeed require hemodynamic studies at the maximal exercise level with measurements of the maximal cardiac output and of the maximal $a\text{-}\bar{v}_{O2}$ difference. To our knowledge such data have never been reported and we

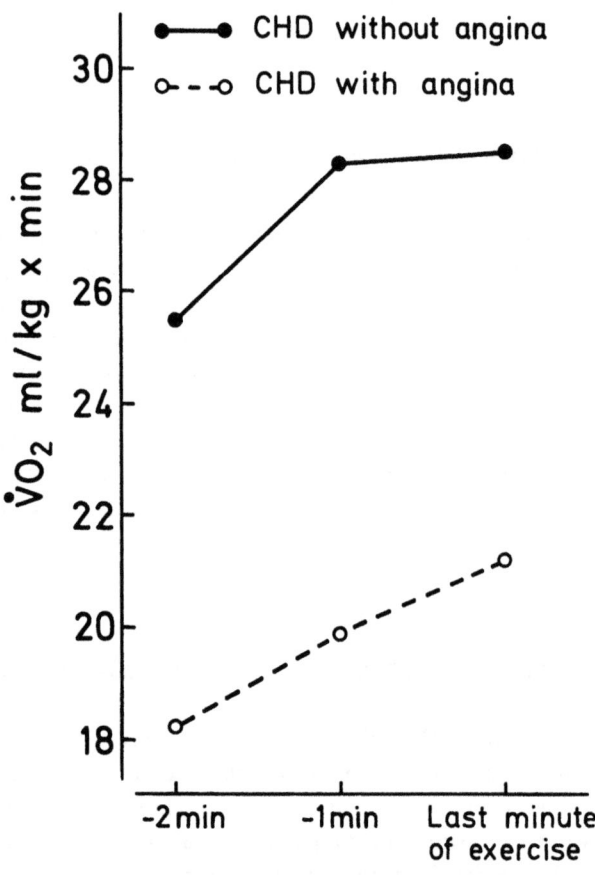

Fig. 12. — Oxygen consumption during the last 3 minutes of the Bruce's multistage treadmill test in 19 patients with coronary heart disease (CHD) but no angina pectoris and in 27 angina patients (from Detry and Bruce, 1971a).

are therefore obliged to rely on predicted or calculated maximal values. The present section will focus on patients with healed myocardial infarction (no angina pectoris) but no clinical signs of heart failure at rest.

1. Maximal heart rate.

The maximal heart rate of coronary patients without angina pectoris appears to be slightly lower than for control subjects of the same age (table 12); Kasser and Bruce (1969) also reported that the maximal heart rate of 28 patients with healed myocardial infarction was 19 beats lower (155 versus 174) than in normal healthy subjects. The reason for this possible decrease in maximal heart rate with coronary disease is unknown : in any case it should be stressed that a low maximal heart rate is not a constant finding in coronary patients since it was 174.5 in 6 patients (mean age = 46.5 years) with healed myocardial infarction (Detry et al., 1971). Interestingly, Benestad (1968) mentioned that the maximal heart rate of coronary patients was closer to the expected normal values when a plateau in oxygen consumption was clearly demonstrated ; it is not known whether the low values of maximal heart rate published by Kasser and Bruce (1969) result from inclusion of patients who did not present a levelling-off of the O_2 consumption.

2. Cardiac output.

Hemodynamic responses of coronary patients without angina pectoris at submaximal exercise levels have been variously assessed. According to several authors the relation of cardiac output to oxygen consumption during submaximal exercise is not altered in coronary patients (Chapman and Fraser, 1954 ; Malmcroma et al., 1963 ; Follath, 1966 ; Clausen et al., 1969). Cardiac outputs measured during submaximal exercise in 12 coronary patients are presented in relation to oxygen consumption in fig. 13 (Detry et al., 1971); the data of coronary patients without angina pectoris were similar to those of angina patients and they did not differ from those collected in normal sedentary middle aged men (Hartley et al., 1969). Other studies indicate, however, that during exercise, cardiac outputs of coronary patients are lower than those of control subjects (Messer et al., 1963 ; Cohen et al., 1965 ; Malmborg, 1965) but all these reports include a large percentage of angina patients in whom the cardiac output was measured during anginal pain precipitated by exercise. At a given absolute level of exercise,

patients developing angina pectoris usually have a lower stroke volume and a lower cardiac output than coronary patients without angina pectoris (Malmcroma et al., 1963 ; Cohen et al., 1965 ; Parker et al., 1967); inclusion of patients studied during anginal pain can therefore account partly for the lower cardiac output.

3. Filling pressure of the left ventricle.

Coronary patients without clinical signs of heart failure at rest often present during submaximal exercise an abnormal elevation of the left ventricular end-diastolic pressure, pulmonary capillary pressure and mean pulmonary arterial pressure which reflect acute left ventricular failure and/or altered compliance of the left ventricle (Müller and Rorvik, 1958 ;Malmborg, 1965). Although such elevation of the left ventricular filling pressure is more often noted in angina patients it is also present in many

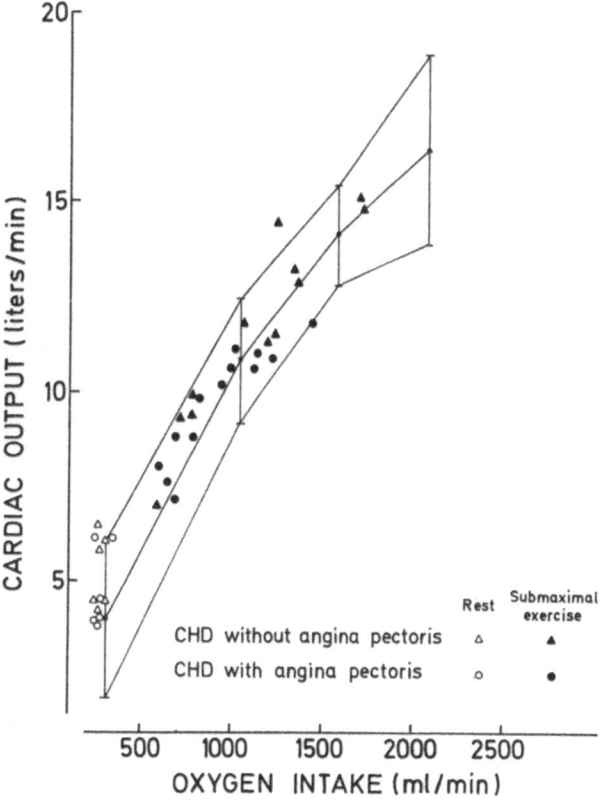

Fig. 13. — Cardiac output in relation to oxygen intake at rest and during submaximal exercise in upright posture in 12 sedentary patients (mean age = 47.8 years) with coronary heart disease - CHD - (from Detry et al., 1971). The lines (mean value ± 1 standard deviation) denote the relationship between cardiac output and oxygen intake in 13 middle-aged (mean age = 47 years) healthy men (Hartley et al., 1969).

patients without angina pectoris (Malmborg, 1965 ; Parker et al., 1967). When the pressure is measured only in the mean pulmonary artery, one should consider the total pulmonary resistance which does not increase during exercise in healthy subjects (Kremer et al., 1967). These abnormal pressure responses at submaximal exercise can be prevented in most patients by sublingual nitroglycerin (Müller and Rorvik, 1958 ; Parker et al., 1967) or by acute digitalization (Malmborg, 1965). It can be logically postulated that transient left ventricular failure is more likely to occur at the maximal exercise level and that it is an important factor in the functional impairment of patients without angina ; experimental data to support this hypothesis are, however, still lacking. The small increase in $V_{O2,max}$ presented by patients with healed myocardial infarction after sublingual nitroglycerin might result partly from a decrease in the left ventricular end-diastolic pressure during exercise (Detry and Bruce, 1971a).

4. Stroke volume.

A characteristic common to all coronary patients is their low stroke volume at rest and during exercise; in patients without angina pectoris this low stroke volume is often attended by a higher heart rate and the cardiac output is then similar to that of control subjects (Malmcroma et al., 1963 ; Follath, 1967 ; Detry et al., 1971). Impaired stroke volume is probably the result of reduced myocardial contractility due to chronic myocardial ischemia and/or to myocardial fibrosis secondary to prior myocardial infarction ; the exact role of ventricular zones which become hypokinetic or akinetic during myocardial ischemia should also be considered (Dwyer, 1970 ;

Lichtlen, 1970). While normal subjects are able to maintain a constant stroke volume during exercise of increasing severity up to the maximal exercise level, the stroke volume of coronary patients often tends to decrease when the severity of exercise increases (fig. 14) ; this trend exists in all coronary patients whether or not limited by angina pectoris (Detry et al., 1971). This inability to maintain the maximal stroke volume at high levels of exercise may reflect incipient heart failure when the myocardial stress increases.

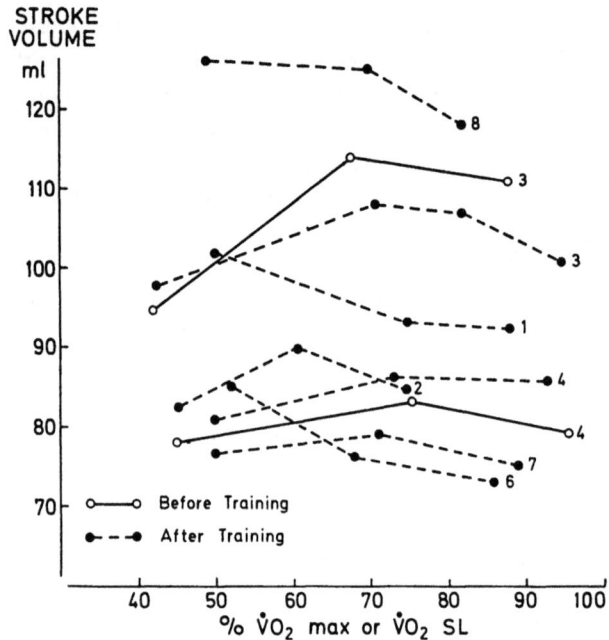

Fig. 14. — Stroke volume during submaximal exercise in relation to the % of the $V_{O2,max}$ or the $V_{O2,SL}$ in coronary patients. The number at the end of each line refers to the number of the patients in Detry et al. (1971).

TABLE 13

Measured and calculated data at the maximal exercise level in 4 coronary patients without angina pectoris (subjects n_o 4, 5, 6 and 8 in Detry et al., 1971).

	$V_{O2,max}$ ml/kg.min	$V_{O2,max}$ ml/min	Maximal HR beats/min	Qs at 70 % of $V_{O2,max}$ ml/beat	Calculated maximal Q l/min	Calculated maximal $a-\bar{v}_{O2}$ diff. ml/100 ml
Before physical training	29.38	2.148	179	92.5	16.6	12.8
After physical training	33.31	2.399	177	93.2	16.4	14.6
Abbreviations : HR = Heart Rate ; Qs = Stroke Volume ; Q = Cardiac Output.						

5. Calculated maximal hemodynamic data.

In 4 sedentary patients with coronary heart disease but no angina pectoris, the maximal cardiac output calculated as the product of measured maximal heart rate (multistage treadmill test) and stroke volume measured at an exercise level corresponding to 75 % of the $\dot{V}_{O2,max}$ averaged 16.6 l/min (Detry et al., 1971); from this calculated maximal cardiac output one can estimate the maximal a-$\bar{v}_{O2}$ difference at 12.8 ml/100 ml, which is a surprisingly low value (table 13). These calculations suggest that patients with healed myocardial infarction have a lower maximal a-$\bar{v}_{O2}$ difference than sedentary healthy subjects : this lower a-v_{O2} difference may perhaps be related to excessive inactivity due to the disease since after 3 months of physical training the calculated maximal a-$\bar{v}_{O2}$ difference had reached values close to those of healthy controls (table 13). These calculations have to be interpreted with great caution, however, since they are based on the assumption that stroke volume does not decrease at the maximal exercise level, which is probably not true (fig. 14); if it is assumed that before training the stroke volume at maximal exercise is only 10 % lower than at 75 % of the $\dot{V}_{O2,max}$, than the calculated a-$\bar{v}_{O2}$ difference at maximal exercise level would increase from 12.8 to 14.3. It is therefore concluded that hemodynamic studies at the maximal exercise level are needed to permit an accurate analysis of the factors limiting the physical work capacity of these patients.

B. Coronary patients with angina pectoris.

The physical work capacity of angina patients is limited by the onset of anginal pain which forces the patients to interrupt exercise. As demonstrated in figure 12, the oxygen consumption measured at the maximal exercise level in angina patients is a symptom limited one and does not fulfill the criteria for $\dot{V}_{O2,max}$. Numerous clinical studies in recent years have been bevoted to the pathophysiology of angina pectoris and to the factors likely to modify the angina threshold ; these studies have permitted a more comprehensive approach of the evaluation and the treatment of angina patients (Mason et al., 1969 ; Piette et al., 1970 ; Epstein et al., 1971).

1. Pathophysiology of angina pectoris.

a) Exertional angina pectoris.

Angina pectoris with exertion is a syndrome reflecting an acute imbalace between the myocardial oxygen requirements and the oxygen supply to the myocardium restricted by diseased coronary arteries. Robinson B. (1967) demonstrated that in a given patient, angina pectoris precipitated by exercise occured at a fixed and reproducible value of the product of heart rate and systolic blood pressure, corrected when necessary for changes in ejection time (triple product); his conclusions were later confirmed by several studies (Balcon et al., 1968 ; Piette et al., 1970 ; Redwood et al., 1971). The protocol of the exercise test is important for the determination of the triple product at the onset of angina ; the exercise test should start at a low level since the use of supramaximal workloads cause an overestimation of the angina threshold (Redwood et al., 1971).

Anginal pain precipitated by exercise is often attended by an increase in left ventricular filling pressure (Müller and Rorvik, 1958). At a similar absolute exercise level, the left ventricular end-diastolic pressure is usually higher in patients experiencing angina pectoris than in patients remaining free of pain while the stroke volume is lower (Parker et al., 1966, 1967). The increase in the filling pressure of the left ventricle occurs before anginal pain is experienced, however, and it is not a constant finding (Müller and Rorvik, 1958 ; Cohen et al., 1965 ; Malmborg, 1965); this usually greater elevation of the left ventricular end-diastolic pressure during angina pectoris probably indicates greater depression of the left ventricular function due to more severe myocardial ischemia during anginal pain. Elevated end-diastolic pressure of the left ventricle may explain the high incidence of atrial gallop sounds recorded after exercise in angina patients (Aronow et al., 1971c).

Although the role of the factors altering the balance between myocardial oxygen demand and supply in the determination of the exercise anginal threshold is increasingly clear, the mechanisms or the substances actually causing the pain are not known (Sampson and Cheitlin, 1971).

b) Pacing-induced angina pectoris.

When anginal pain is precipitated by atrial pacing, there is also in most subjects a fixed relationship between the angina threshold and the tension-time index or the triple product (Sowton et al., 1967 ; Frick et al., 1968). The heart volume, which is not taken into account in the indices reflecting the myocardial oxygen requirements, is also important ; acute increase or decrease of circulating blood volume and presumably heart volume during atrial pacing modify indeed the angina threshold (Parker et al., 1970a ; Khaja et al., 1971). During atrial pacing in coronary patients, the cardiac output does not change significantly, the heart volume decreases and the ejection period is shortened ; the left ventricular end-diastolic pressure decreases in patients without angina pectoris but not when anginal pain is precipitated (Sowton et al., 1967 ; O'Brien et al., 1969 ; Parker et al., 1969a). Accordingly, one would expect anginal pain with atrial pacing to occur at higher values of tension-time index than when induced by exercise ; Balcon et al. (1969) reported, however, that the tension-time index at the level of pain was the same, whether induced by supine exercise or atrial pacing, while O'Brien et al. (1969) pointed out that anginal pain with atrial pacing occurred at a significantly lower tension-time index than with exercise. These unexplained findings need to be confirmed, however.

Unchanged left ventricular end-diastolic pressure during pacing induced angina represents in fact an abnormal response to pacing and the left ventricular function curve is shifted to the right, which indicates a depressed left ventricular function during angina pectoris (Parker et al., 1969a ; Dwyer, 1970). The depression of the left ventricular function during angina is attended by a decreased left ventricular compliance as demonstrated by Dwyer (1970); this author also pointed out that acute myocardial ischemia induced by atrial pacing often caused reversible regional disorders of the left ventricular contraction, i.e. the appearance of hypokinetic or akinetic zones. The role of asygerny of the left ventricular contraction in the determination of the anginal treshold remains to be established, however.

When atrial pacing is prolonged after the onset of anginal pain, Shappell et al. (1970) have observed a progressive increase in the P_{50}(*) of the coronary sinus blood, i.e. a decrease in hemoglobin affinity for oxygen ; this acute rightward shift in oxyhemoglobin dissociation curve increases the delivery of oxygen to the myocardium without any associated change in coronary blood flow or in tissue P_{O_2}. This transient change in hemoglobin affinity for oxygen during anginal pain is not attended by increased erythrocytic 2-3 diphosphoglycerate levels, and no mediating factor has yet been identified (Mulhausen, 1970 ; Shappell et al., 1970). Abnormal oxyhemoglobin dissociation curve, with P_{50} greater

than normal, have been reported by Eliot and Bratt (1969) in young women with previous myocardial necrosis but normal coronary arteriograms ; although these findings, namely a rightward shift in the oxyhemoglobin dissociation curve, should facilitate the delivery of oxygen to the myocardium, surprisingly these authors speculated about a possible causal relationship between abnormal release of oxygen by hemoglobin and unexplained myocardial necrosis.

c) *Spontaneous angina pectoris.*

Prinzmetal's variant angina pectoris presents several typical features : the pain occurs at rest or during mild exertion usually at about the same time of the day, it is more severe than the classical exertional angina pectoris and the electrocardiogram shows elevations of the ST segment (Prinzmetal et al., 1960). In 3 out of 4 patients with this syndrome, spontaneous ST segment elevation has been recorded in the absence of any pain and it is not known whether the factors causing the pain and the ST segment elevation are identical (Guazzi et al., 1970). These spontaneous anginal episodes are not caused by elevation of heart rate or blood pressure and they are attended by a depression of the left ventricular function with systemic hypotension and a decreased cardiac output (Guazzi et al., 1971). This syndrome is often associated with a narrowing of an important coronary vessel and it has been suggested that the pain was caused by a coronary spasm ; complete occlusion of the diseased coronary artery with a resulting myocardial infarction can lead to the disappearance of the anginal syndrome (Prinzmetal et al., 1960) but this is not constant (Guazzi et al., 1970). The theory according to which these spontaneous anginal episodes are caused by a constriction of a coronary vessel is tempting but has not yet received experimental support ; such spasm of the coronary arteries have been demonstrated angiographically (Proudfit et al., 1966) but a possible constricting effect of the contrast medium cannot be eliminated.

Spontaneous angina pectoris described by Roughgarden (1966) is different from Prinzmetal's variant angina pectoris since it is usually preceded by an elevation of the systemic arterial pressure and not systematically attended by ST segment elevation ; Rosland (1969) also mentioned that the pressure-rate product at the onset of spontaneous angina

---

(*) P_{50} is the oxygen partial pressure at 50 % oxygen saturation

varied from one crisis to another. This type of angina is therefore intermediate between the exertional angina pectoris and Prinzmetal's variant form.

2. Factors modifying the anginal threshold.

The factors which modify the hemodynamic response to exercise also influence the physical work capacity of angina patients.

When exercised in a *cool environment*, angina patients may experience angina pectoris at an exercise level which does not cause the pain in a warmer environment : this worsening of the symptoms is due to a greater pressure response when exercise is performed at a reduced environmental temperature (Epstein et al., 1969).

Postprandial angina pectoris is caused by a less severe exercise than under control conditions ; the triple product at the onset of angina pectoris is not modified following a meal, however, and the lower physical capacity of angina patients is therefore due to greater heart rate and systolic pressure responses when exercise is performed after a meal (Goldstein et al., 1971b).

Exercise tolerance of angina patients is decreased by *cigarette smoking* ; this adverse effect of smoking results from higher heart rate and blood pressure responses to submaximal exercise due to nicotine and from an increased carboxy-hemoglobin level (Aronow et al., 1971b). The pressure-rate product at the onset of angina pectoris is decreased by smoking non-nicotine cigarettes, although these do not modify the heart rate and blood pressure responses to exercise ; this has been attributed to the high carboxy-hemoglobin level which reduces the amount of oxygen deliverable to the myocardium (Aronow and Rokaw, 1971).

Emotional angina pectoris appears to be due to the hemodynamic stress attending emotion since the triple product at the onset of such angina was the same as for angina pectoris precipitated by exercise (Robinson B., 1967).

Nitroglycerin increases exercise tolerance of angina patients ; in 32 patients with angina pectoris, $\dot{V}_{O_2,SL}$ in fact increased 14.5 % with sublingual nitroglycerin (Detry and Bruce, 1971a). In a large percentage of patients (30 to 39 %) sublingual nitroglycerin or isosorbide-dinitrate also prevents anginal pain so that physical work capacity is no longer limited by anginal pain but rather by fatigue or dyspnea (Detry and Bruce, 1971a ; Goldstein et al., 1971a). The mechanisms of action of nitroglycerin in angina patients are still somewhat discussed.

After sublingual nitroglycerin (table 9), the maximal pressure-rate product appears to be higher in angina patients (Robinson, 1968 ; Detry and Bruce, 1971a ; Goldstein et al., 1971a); the values reported by Goldstein et al. (1971a) in fact underestimate the increase in maximal pressure-rate product after nitroglycerin, since these researchers excluded from their figures all patients (39 %) in whom angina pectoris was prevented. After nitroglycerin, the ejection time is decreased so that the corrected pressure-rate product (triple product) at the maximal exercise level is not modified (Robinson, 1968 ; Goldstein et al., 1971a); the validity of correcting the pressure-rate product for the ejection time can be questioned, however, (Monroe, 1964). Parker et al. (1966) reported that in 11 out of 14 angina patients, exertional anginal pain was prevented by sublingual nitroglycerin without any modification in the tension-time index (which also accounts for possible variations in ejection time) and they attributed this preventive action of the drug to a decrease in heart volume. A lower heart volume during post-nitroglycerin exercise has been recently demonstrated by Goldstein et al. (1971a) and is likely to result from the action of the drug on the peripheral venous bed, namely an increased venous compliance causing peripheral venous pooling of blood (Detry et al., 1972b). Reduced heart volume with nitroglycerin diminishes the myocardial oxygen requirements for a given pressure-rate product and may therefore account for the greater pressure-rate product repeatedly observed at maximal exercise in angina patients treated with nitroglycerin.

Another major effect of nitroglycerin in angina patients is to decrease the filling pressure of the left ventricle during exercise (Müller and Rorvik, 1958 ; Parker et al., 1966 ; Najmi et al., 1967 ; Arborelius et al., 1968 ; Wiener et al., 1969); this action goes along with an improvement of the left ventricular function and reflects lower myocardial ischemia probably resulting from reduced heart volume (Parker et al., 1966). Angina pectoris precipitated by atrial pacing is usually prevented by nitroglycerin which also improves the left ventricular function (Parker et al., 1969a) ; these effects of nitroglycerin are very similar to those of phlebotomy. Parker et al. (1970a) demonstrated indeed that an acute decrease in circulating blood volume caused the disappearance of anginal pain induced by pacing without any change in tension-time index ; restoration of blood volume by reinfusion of blood caused the reappearance of anginal pain without further changes in tension-time index. These data of Parker et al. (1970a) strongly suggest that peripheral venous pooling of blood with a consequent decrease in heart volume is an important mechanism in the action of nitroglycerin on the anginal threshold. As already mentioned in chapter 2, a redistribution of coronary blood flow with nitroglycerin could also play a role in the improvement of angina patients (Becker et al., 1971).

Beta-blocking agents acutely modify the angina threshold since after beta-blockade, angina pectoris occurs at significantly lower values of pressure-rate product (see chapter 2).

Digitalis improved exercise tolerance of approximately 50 % of the angina patients studied by Malmborg (1965); this prevention of the anginal pain was usually associated with a decrease of the intracardiac pressures. As pointed out in chapter I, the effects of digitalis on the angina threshold depend on a balance between the effects on heart volume and those on myocardial contractility (Sonnenblick et al., 1968 ; Braunwald, 1971); one should therefore expect digitalis to be more effective in patients with enlarged heart volume and hemodynamic signs of left ventricular failure with exertion. On the other hand, increased myocardial contractility in those patients with normal heart volume can lead to a worsening of the symptoms.

Carotid sinus nerve stimulation has been proposed for the treatment of refractory angina pectoris by Braunwald et al., (1967b); stimulation of the carotid sinus nerve during exercise causes a decrease in heart rate and blood pressure which account for the increased exercise tolerance of angina patients. The angina threshold is not modified by this therapy, however, since the pressure-rate product at the onset of pain is similar with or without carotid sinus nerve stimulation (Epstein et al., 1971).

The effects of *physical training* on the anginal threshold will be discussed in chapter 4.

CHAPTER IV

Physical training in coronary heart disease

The increasing incidence of coronary heart disease in the middle-aged population and the decrease in mortality in the early stages of acute myocardial infarction set imperiously the problem of the rehabilitation of coronary patients. A few years ago, prolonged bed rest and abstention from physical activity were still commonly recommended to patients recovering from acute myocardial infarction ; overcaution among general practitioners and cardiologists combined with the patient's fear and a protective familial environment often resulted in chronic invalidism. Numerous recent studies have demonstrated the fallacy of such a therapeutic approach and indicated that most patients with coronary heart disease could return to a productive and enjoyable life ; many studies have also pointed out that physical activity was not harmful to patients with steady coronary heart disease and

that supervised physical training led to significant physical and psychological benefits.

The rehabilitation of coronary patients includes several steps from the onset of symptoms to the return to full-time employment or maximum advisable activity ; during this period, all aspects of the disease have to be considered and treated adequately. This chapter will focus on one aspect of the rehabilitation of coronary patients, namely the physical training of patients with a previous myocardial infarction and/or exertional angina pectoris. The effects of physical training in coronary patients will be compared to the results of physical training of healthy sedentary subjects ; since athletes represent an extremely well trained fraction of the population, it is of interest to review first the physiological characteristics of athletes.

PHYSIOLOGICAL CHARACTERISTICS OF ATHLETES

Athletes differ from sedentary or unfit persons by their exceptional capacity to perform very heavy exercises for short or long periods of time. This performance capacity depends on numerous factors, including the energy production from aerobic and anaerobic processes, the neuromuscular function and psychological factors such as motivation and tactics (Saltin and Åstrand, 1967 ; Åstrand, and Rodahl, 1970); these factors play different roles in different sports. Energy output from aerobic processes is essential in endurance events athletes, who are characterized by very high $V_{O2,max}$; in sports events requiring short-time performances, the role of anaerobic processes is more important, as indicated by the relatively lower $V_{O2,max}$ measured in weightlifters for instance (Roskamm, 1967 ; Saltin and Åstrand, 1967). We will limit our brief analysis to the factors determining the physical capacity of athletes in endurance events.

A. Maximal cardiac output.

Athletes in endurance events have very high $V_{O2,max}$; the highest individual values reported are 6.24 l/min (Ekblom and Hermansen, 1968) and 85.1 ml/kg min (Saltin and Åstrand, 1967). These $V_{O2,max}$ result essentially from high maximal cardiac output entirely due to high stroke volumes (table 14) since the maximal heart rate of athletes tends to be slightly lower than that of sedentary persons (Lester et al., 1968). The most fit athletes are characterized by the highest stroke volumes and top international athletes differ from those of regional class by their greater maximal stroke volume (Ekblom and Hermansen, 1968). The $V_{O2,max}$ of athletes is therefore largely determined by their maximal stroke volume and there is a close linear relationship between the $V_{O2,max}$ and the maximal stroke volume ; the coefficient of correlation between these 2 parameters was 0.93 in a group of 25 young well trained male subjects (Åstrand, et al., 1964 ; Ekblom and Hermansen, 1968).

TABLE 14

Hemodynamic determinants of $\dot{V}_{O2,max}$ in young male athletes (from Ekblom and Hermansen, 1968).

Number of subjects	Age years	$\dot{V}_{O2,max}$		HR beats/min	Qs ml/beat	Q l/min	$a\text{-}v_{O2}$ diff. ml/100 ml
		l/min	ml/kg.min				
8 *	26.3	5.57	73.9	190	189	36.0	15.6
5 **	24.6	4.58	64.2	191	149	28.4	16.1

* Athletes of international class.   ** Athletes of regional class.

Abbreviations : *HR* = Heart Rate ; *Qs* = Stroke Volume ; *Q* = Cardiac Output.

B. Maximal arterio-venous oxygen difference.

The maximal $a\text{-}v_{O2}$ difference of young athletes varies between 15.6 and 17.1 (Grimby et al., 1966 ; Ekblom and Hermansen, 1968) and is therefore greater than that of sedentary subjects of similar age (see table 11) ; this difference indicates mostly a greater extraction of oxygen by the working muscles during maximal exercise and also perhaps a more complete redistribution of the maximal cardiac output. At the maximal exercise level, the muscle blood flows (per g of muscle) of athletes and untrained subjects are similar (Grimby et al., 1967) : the higher maximal cardiac output of athletes should therefore result essentially from their greater working muscle mass during maximal exercise.

C. Dimensions of the oxygen transport system.

High $\dot{V}_{O2,max}$ of athletes are attended by large dimensions of the oxygen transport system : the vital capacity, the red cell volume and the total hemoglobin are indeed higher in athletes who are also characterized by large heart volumes (Reindell et al., 1967 ; Åstrand and Rodahl, 1970). The heart volume is linearly related to the maximal stroke volume and to the $\dot{V}_{O2,max}$ but these relationships are not very close because of a wide dispersion of individual values (Åstrand et al., 1964 ; Roskamm, 1967); Ekblom and Hermansen (1968) reported indeed data on 2 top athletes having the same $\dot{V}_{O2,max}$ (5.6 l/min) and the same maximal stroke volume (182 ml/beat) but heart volumes of 950 and 1290 ml respectively. Accordingly, the stroke volume of athletes does not depend only on the dimensions of the heart but also on the contractile force of the left ventricle which determines the ejection fraction (ratio of stroke volume and left ventricular end-diastolic volume).

The high physical work capacity of athletes is determined by many factors. Very hard and regular physical training is obviously essential in order to achieve and maintain high performance capacity ; many athletes began their training during adolescence and this early training appears very important since it induces a greater development of the oxygen transport system (Åstrand, et al., 1963 ; Ekblom, 1969). Genetic factors, still to be identified, probably also play a major role, mostly in those athletes reaching top international class (Åstrand and Rodahl, 1970). Continuous training is also essential to maintain a high performance level and sedentarity or a short bed rest period cause a sharp decrease in the physical work capacity of athletes (Saltin et al., 1968).

D. Effects of aging.

As in sedentary subjects, the $\dot{V}_{O2,max}$ of athletes decreases with age ; this decrease in $\dot{V}_{O2,max}$ results from the physiological decrease of the maximal heart rate with age (Lester et al., 1968) and also from a lower maximal $a\text{-}v_{O2}$ difference in older athletes. In 9 middle-aged (mean age = 51 years) but still active athletes, the maximal $a\text{-}v_{O2}$ difference was indeed only 13.3 ml/100 ml (Grimby et al., 1966); this lower maximal $a\text{-}v_{O2}$ difference does not result from lower blood hemoglobin level since it was at rest the same (13.5 g/100 ml) as in the young athletes studied by Ekblom and Hermansen (1968). These data suggest lower peripheral oxygen extraction by the working muscles in older athletes. The evolution of the maximal stroke volume of athletes with age has still to be determined since comparisons of cross-sectional studies suggest either no change or a decrease in the stroke volume with aging (Grimby et al., 1966 ; Ekblom and Hermansen, 1968).

E. Former athletes.

Middle-aged athletes who have discontinued training for many years have lower $\dot{V}_{O2,max}$ than still active athletes of the same age, but their $V_{O2,max}$ is higher than that of sedentary subjects ; interestingly the heart volume of former athletes is not different from that of still active athletes (Pyörälä et al., 1967 ; Saltin and Grimby, 1968). Former athletes, even if now sedentary, therefore keep some charac- teristics of well trained athletes as a consequence of their earlier training and/or of constitutional factors ; on the other hand, continuous training of athletes can partly prevent the physiological decrease of $V_{O2,max}$ with aging.

PHYSICAL TRAINING OF HEALTHY SEDENTARY SUBJECTS

Physical training of sedentary subjects increases their physical work capacity and modifies their hemodynamic response to submaximal and maximal exercise. In this section we will review the few longitudinal studies including measured data at the maximal exercise level before and after a period of physical training ; the factors influencing the response to physical training and the mechanisms of action of physical training will be discussed.

A. Maximal oxygen intake.

In most centers, the physical reconditioning programs consist of 2 or 3 weekly sessions, each session lasting 45 to 60 minutes ; in a few months such programs cause a significant increase in the $V_{O2,max}$, ranging from 10 to 20 % (table 15). This response to training is influenced by several factors.

1. Initial level of physical fitness.

The initial level of physical fitness is important since in a given age group, the most important increases in $V_{O2,max}$ (expressed in % of initial values) are measured in the subjects with the lowest initial $V_{O2,max}$; this finding means that the most spectacular results of physical training will be encountered in the most sedentary subjects (Saltin et al., 1968 ; Kiblom, 1971). When sedentarity is prescribed, as with forced complete bed rest for a few weeks, the increase in $V_{O2,max}$ with physical training can reach 96 % (Saltin et al., 1968).

2. Intensity of physical training.

The intensity of the physical training also plays a major role in the determination of the results since training at too low an intensity does not cause any increase in the physical work capacity (Roskamm, 1967). In young subjects, the heart rate during physical training must be above 135 beats/min to induce significant changes in the $V_{O2,max}$ (Roskamm, 1967). In middle-aged or old subjects, who have a lower maximal heart rate, the intensity of the training programs is usually adjusted so that the heart rate during training equals the resting heart rate plus 70 % of the difference between the maximal heart rate and the resting heart rate (Roskamm, 1967 ; Kiblom, 1971). In some centers, the physical training program is entirely submaximal (Siegel et al., 1970 ; Kiblom, 1971) while others include some periods of maximal exercise in the program (Rowell, 1962 ; Ekblom et al., 1968 ; Saltin et al., 1968, 1969); these differences have to be kept in mind in the analysis of the data presented in table 15. The lower increase in $V_{O2,max}$ in the women studied by Kiblom (1971) probably results from the lower intensity of the training program. The large improvement reported by Siegel et al. (1970) is probably due to the extreme sedentarity of the subjects who were all blind. The training program used by Siegel et al. (1970) was very light since each session included only 12 minutes of submaximal bicycle exercise ; it is doubtful whether so light a program would be as effective in less sedentary subjects (Roskamm, 1967). Once the physical work capacity has increased as the result of physical training, it is essential to continue to train regularly in order to maintain the benefits (Roskamm, 1967); Siegel et al. (1970) reported that a weekly session of 12 minutes was not sufficient to maintain the $V_{O2,max}$ at the level achieved by more frequent training.

3. Influence of age and sex.

The influence of age on the effects of physical training has still to be firmly established. The percent increase in $V_{O2,max}$ with training did not vary with age in the male subjects studied by Saltin et al. (1969) while it tended to be lower in the older subjects of both sexes studied by others (Roskamm, 1967 ; Kiblom, 1971). In older subjects, physical training often causes complications such as tendinitis,

TABLE 15

Effects of physical training on the $\dot{V}_{O_2,max}$ in sedentary healthy subjects.

Source	Number of subjects	Sex	Age years	Intensity of training *	$\dot{V}_{O_2,max}$ l/min and ml/kg.min**		
					Before	After	% change
Saltin, 1969 ***	17	M	21.6	++	3.11 44.6	3.59 51.6	+ 15.4 + 15.6
Saltin et al., 1969	42	M	40.5	++	2.89 37.5	3.44 44.3	+ 19.0 + 18.1
Naughton and Nagle, 1965	18	M	40	+(?)	— 31.3	— 36.8	— + 17.6
Siegel et al., 1970	9	M	46	+	1.63 24.0	1.94 28.5	+ 19.0 + 18.7
Saltin et al., 1969	8	M	55.3	++	2.25 28.0	2.67 33.3	+ 18.7 + 18.9
Kiblom, 1971	12	F	23.7	+	1.94 36.8	2.18 40.8	+ 12.4 + 10.9
	8	F	44.0	+	1.98 31.0	2.20 35.1	+ 11.1 + 13.2
	13	F	56.4	+	1.66 26.9	1.80 29.4	+ 8.4 + 9.3

* + = training at submaximal intensity ; ++ = training including periods at the maximal exercise level.

** $\dot{V}_{O_2,max}$ in liter/min (first horizontal line) and in ml/kg.min (second horizontal line).

*** From data of Rowell (1962) ; Ekblom et al. (1968) and Saltin et al. (1968).

TABLE 16

Effects of physical training on the hemodynamic determinants of the $\dot{V}_{O_2,max}$ in healthy sedentary subjects, expressed as percent changes ·from pre-training values.

Sources	Number of subjects	Age years	Sex	$\dot{V}_{O_2}$ l/min	HR beats/min	Qs ml/beat	Q l/min	a-v_{O_2} diff. ml/100 ml
Saltin, 1969	17	21.6	M	+ 15	— 3	+ 11	+ 8	+ 8
Hartley et al., 1969	13	47	M	+ 14	— 3	+ 16	+ 13	+ 1
Kiblom and Astrand, 1971	9	33	F	+ 10.3	— 0.5	+ 11.5	+ 10.5	— 0.7
	4	55	F	+ 6.3	+ 2.4	+ 5.8	+ 8.7	— 5.1

Abbreviations : HR = Heart Rate ; Qs = Stroke Volume ; Q = Cardiac Output.

sprains or muscle injuries, which some time require the interruption of the program : great care should therefore always be taken with old subjects, particularly at the beginning of a physical training program (Kiblom et al., 1969 ; Mann et al., 1969 ; Grimby and Saltin, 1971). The fear of such complications, occurring essentially with calisthenics, jogging or running, led Kiblom (1971) to train her subjects on a bicycle ergometer.

The sex does not appear to influence the results of physical training (Roskamm, 1967) and, as stated above, the lower improvement noted in women by Kiblom (1971) is probably due to the lower intensity of the training program.

B. Hemodynamic responses at the maximal exercise level.

The increase in $V_{O2,max}$ with physical training is due to changes in its hemodynamic determinants. The results of the few studies including hemodynamic data at the maximal exercise level are presented in table 16 (Rowell, 1962 ; Ekblom et al., 1968 ; Saltin et al., 1968 ; Hartley et al., 1969 ; Kiblom and Åstrand, 1971). In young male subjects the 15 % increase in $V_{O2,max}$ with physical training is produced by an increase in both the maximal a-$\bar{v}_{O2}$ difference (+ 8 %) and the maximal cardiac output (+ 8 %) due to greater stroke volume. The 14 % increase in $V_{O2,max}$ noted in sedentary middle-aged men results entirely from a greater maximal cardiac output (+ 13 %) and maximal stroke volume (+ 16 %) after physical training : the reason why the maximal a-v_{O2} difference is not modified with training in middle-aged men is unknown. The results reported by Kiblom and Åstrand (1971) in young and older women are similar to those obtained in middle-aged men, i.e. the increase in $V_{O2,max}$ results from a greater maximal cardiac output. Since the training followed by the women was less intense than that followed by the men presented in table 16, one may question whether the lack of increase in maximal a-$\bar{v}_{O2}$ difference with training in the young women is not simply due to the lower intensity of the training program. The maximal muscle blood flow (per 100 g of muscle) of trained and untrained subjects is similar and the increase in maximal cardiac output always noted after training in sedentary subjects should consequently reflect a greater working muscle mass at maximal exercise after physical conditioning (Grimby et al., 1967).

C. Submaximal exercise data.

Physical training constantly reduces the heart rate at rest and at submaximal exercise levels ; the blood pressure also tends to decrease and the myocardial oxygen requirements are probably lower after training. At a given submaximal exercise level, the oxygen consumption is either unchanged or slightly lower after physical training while the ventilation is usually decreased ; the lactate blood levels are also decreased after training but the relationship between the lactate levels and the relative severity of the exercise is not affected by training.

The effects of physical training on the cardiac output during submaximal exercise are unclear. After training, several authors have measured an unchanged submaximal cardiac output with a higher stroke volume to balance the lower heart rate (Rowell, 1962 ; Frick et al., 1963 ; Saltin et al., 1968 ; Hartley et al., 1969 ; Kiblom and Åstrand, 1971) while others reported a lower cardiac output with a widened a-$\bar{v}_{O2}$ difference (Tabakin et al., 1965 ; Andrew et al., 1966 ; Douglas and Becklake, 1968 ; Ekblom et al., 1968) ; except for the subjects studied by Ekblom et al. (1968), those in whom a lower sub-maximal cardiac output was found after training were not in fact sedentary but rather well trained subjects studied before and after a training season (Tabakin et al., 1965 ; Andrew et al., 1966 ; Douglas and Becklake, 1968).

After training of sedentary subjects, the distribution of the cardiac output at a given submaximal exercise level is probably modified ; the splanchnic and renal blood flow should be greater, since the relative severity of the exercise is lower (Rowell et al., 1964a ; Grimby, 1965), and the muscle blood flow is lower (Varnauskas et al., 1970). This lower muscle blood flow during submaximal exercise after training is attended by an increased activity of the skeletal muscle enzymatic system which may account for an increased oxygen extraction capacity ; numerous studies in animals and humans have indeed demonstrated an increased activity of the muscular respiratory enzymes and an increase in the size and number of the muscle mitochondria after physical conditioning (Holloszy, 1967 ; Gollnick and King, 1969 ; Morgan et al., 1969 ; Short et al., 1970 ; Varnauskas et al., 1970 ; Björntrop et al., 1971 ; Kiessling et al., 1971).

D. Heart volume.

In sedentary subjects the effects of physical training on heart volume are variable but never of great importance. Several studies indicate a slight increase in heart volume after training (Frick et al., 1963 ; Saltin et al., 1968 ; Pyörälä et al., 1971) while in other studies the heart volume did not change (Ekblom et al., 1968 ; Kiblom et al., 1969 ; Kiblom, 1971) or even significantly decreased after training (Siegel et al., 1970). These discrepancies cannot be attributed to differences in the selection of the subjects, their age, their sex, or the intensity of the training. In any case, it is clear that the stroke volume can increase after training without any change in the resting heart volume ; since the resting total heart volume is only a rough index of the left ventricular end-diastolic volume, and no data have been collected during exercise, it is not possible to analyse correctly the mechanisms responsible for the increase in the stroke volume.

E. Mechanisms of action of physical training.

The mechanisms of action of physical training in sedentary normal subjects are not well understood since the data of different investigators are not in complete agreement. According to many authors, physical training essentially increases the maximal cardiac output through an increase in the stroke volume ; this mechanism undoubtedly plays an important role since all studies on sedentary healthy subjects indicate an increased maximal stroke volume after training. It is not known whether this greater stroke volume is produced mostly by an increased left ventricular end-diastolic volume or by increased contractility with a greater left ventricular ejection fraction after training.

The data collected in young sedentary subjects clearly indicate however that physical training can also increase the maximal a-v_{O_2} difference and accordingly the oxygen extraction capacity of the muscles, since a greater redistribution of the maximal cardiac output can account for only a small fraction of this widened maximal a-v_{O_2} difference ; greater peripheral oxygen extraction after training might be directly related to enzymatic changes in the skeletal muscles. It is of interest to mention here that the lower submaximal heart rate after physical training depends at least partly on peripheral adaptation in the working muscles ; Clausen et al. (1970) have indeed reported that bradycardia noted during submaximal leg exercise after physical training with the legs was not present during post-training arm exercise, and reciprocally.

PHYSICAL TRAINING OF CORONARY PATIENTS

Physical training has been used for approximately 10 years in the treatment and rehabilitation of coronary patients and its beneficial effects are now well documented. Before describing the physiological effects of exercise training and analysing its mechanisms of action in patients with coronary heart disease, it is important to review first the methods for exercise training of coronary patients.

A. Methods.

1. Selection of patients.

The selection of the patients should be based on the following principle : physical training is indicated only for patients suffering from a steady and uncomplicated coronary heart disease. Two months should be allowed after a myocardial infarction before the patient may participate to a regular physical training program. In the meantime, the patient will be carefully and progressively mobilized, first passively and then actively ; early rising from bed will also be planned. An early contact between the patient recovering from an acute myocardial infarction and the staff of the rehabilitation center is very important and it will prepare the patient to approach the more active part of the rehabilitation in far better physical and psychological conditions. When the acute stage of myocardial infarction is over, contra-indications to physical training include a refractory heart failure, numerous and multifocal premature ventricular beats or premature ventricular beats precipitated by exercise, a complete atrioventricular block, or a large ventricular aneurysm. Exertional angina pectoris is never in itself a contra-indication to physical training, except when it is evolutive (the so-called preinfarctional angina pectoris). Associated diseases such as diabetes or arterial hypertension are not contra-indications to exercise training when they are successfully controlled.

2. Intensity of physical training.

The intensity of the physical training program will be adjusted to each individual capacity, taking into account the initial physical work capacity, which should always be measured. In coronary patients, the training program will be essentially submaximal; in patients without angina pectoris the training heart rate may be calculated as for normal subjects (training heart rate = resting heart rate + 70 % of the difference between the maximal and the resting heart rate). This calculation is equivalent to choosing a training intensity corresponding to 60 - 70 % of the $\dot{V}_{O_2.max}$ as proposed by Hellerstein and Hornsten (1966). In patients with exertional angina pectoris the intensity of the training will be just below the anginal threshold; these patients should also use nitroglycerin prophylactically. As in healthy subjects, the training program should be progressive and its intensity will be adjusted according to the patient's subjective reaction and feelings and to the results of repeated objective measurements of his physical work capacity. Active supervision of the training program by a well trained professional staff and a physician, who will so remain is close contact with each patient, is finally the best way to determine the proper training intensity. Usually the patients meet 2 or 3 times a week for sessions lasting 45 to 60 minutes.

3. Types of exercises.

The types of exercise used in the training program are not critical as far as they require working with large muscle groups. Some authors use only the bicycle ergometer (Varnauskas et al., 1966; Frick and Katila, 1968; Clausen et al., 1969) while others combine several exercises such as walking, jogging, running, calisthenics, cycling and rowing (Hellerstein and Hornsten, 1966; Naughton et al., 1966; Gottheiner, 1968; Detry et al., 1971; Vandenbroucke, 1971). Isometric exercises causing a disproportionate blood pressure elevation should be avoided at least in angina patients. Each training session begins with a warming up period and ends up with a cooling down period. Whenever possible, the training should be performed in group; group training has obvious practical advantages and it also has excellent psychological effects on the patients; for group training the intensity of the exercises will be adjusted to each patient's capacity as indicated before.

4. Risks of physical training.

The risks of physical training should not be overlooked; Pyfer and Doan (1969) and Bruce and Kluge (1971) have indeed reported 5 cases of cardiac arrest due to ventricular arrhythmias precipitated by exercise training. All these 5 patients responded immediately to a single precordial shock and there were no myocardial infarctions. Accordingly, the physical training sessions should always be under the supervision of a well trained medical and paramedical staff with all resuscitatory equipment at hand.

B. Resting and submaximal exercise data.

1. Heart rate.

All studies on the effects of physical training in coronary patients agree on one point, namely that resting and submaximal heart rate are lower after physical conditioning (Varnauskas et al., 1966; Frick and Katila, 1968; Clausen et al., 1969; Detry et al., 1971; Epstein et al., 1971; Rousseau et al., 1972b). This lower heart rate is attended by a lower systemic arterial pressure (table 17) and lower values of indices of myocardial oxygen requirements such as the pressure-rate product (Hellerstein et al., 1965; Detry et al., 1971; Rousseau et al., 1972b), the triple product (Epstein et al., 1971) and the tension-time index (Frick and Katila, 1968; Clausen et al., 1969). The resting heart volume is not affected by physical training in coronary patients (Frick and Katila, 1968; Clausen et al., 1969; Detry et al., 1971); the effects on myocardial contractility have still to be determined. After training, a coronary patient will therefore perform a given submaximal exercise with presumably lower myocardial oxygen requirements. The submaximal ventilation also decreases after physical training, which accounts for the less frequent shortness of breath in physically conditioned patients.

2. Cardiac output.

The effects of physical training on the submaximal cardiac output are still much debated since the results of the published studies indicate two different possibilities (table 17). According to some authors, the lower post-training heart rate is compensated by an increase in the stroke volume and the cardiac output is not significantly affected by physical training (Clausen et al., 1969; Frick et al., 1971; Rousseau et al., 1972b); others have reported an unchanged stroke volume after physical training with a significant decrease in the submaximal cardiac output (Varnauskas et al., 1966; Detry et al., 1971). Finally, after physical training Clausen and Trap-Jensen (1970) found a decreased cardiac output at a low

TABLE 17

Effects of physical training on the hemodynamic adaptation to submaximal exercise. Comparison with the data collected in a control group. The results are presented as % changes from initial values.

Sources	Number of subjects	$\dot{V}_{O_2}$	HR	Qs	Q	$a\text{-}v_{O_2}$ diff.	$\dot{V}$	Mean arterial pressure	$\dot{V}_{O_2}$**
TRAINING									
Varnauskas et al., 1966	6	+ 1.1	— 5.9	— 6.1	— 10.6*	+ 15.5*	— 1.7	— 6.4	?
Frick et al., 1971	10	— 1.7	— 7.5*	+ 9.3*	+ 2.1	— 3.2	—	+ 2.5	1316
Clausen et al., 1969	7	— 0.6	— 8.0*	+ 7.1	— 0.4	+ 1.0	— 11.1*	— 14.3*	1251
Clausen and Trap-Jensen, 1970	6	— 1.5	— 13.5*	+ 0.5	— 14.0*	+ 13.5	— 10.0*	— 12.5*	1070
	6	— 2.0	— 9.0*	+ 14.0*	+ 5.5	— 7.0	— 13.0*	— 14.5*	1475
Detry et al., 1971	10	— 5.5	— 14.5*	+ 1.0	—13.0*	+ 9.0*	— 16.0*	— 5.5*	771
	11	— 2.0	— 11.5*	+ 2.0	— 9.0*	+ 8.5*	— 14.0*	— 7.0*	1283
Rousseau et al., 1972	16	— 3.6	— 13.3*	+ 10.7*	— 4.2	+ 1.5	— 7.3*	— 3.2	685
	20	— 2.8*	— 15.6*	+ 14.9*	— 3.4	+ 1.0	— 13.5*	— 3.9	1077
	11	— 1.3	— 14.5*	+ 18.3*	— 0.8	+ 0.1	— 13.6*	— 1.8	1392
CONTROLS									
Bergman and Varnauskas, 1971	10	—	— 8.3*	—	—	—	—	—	—
Frick et al., 1971	4	+ 0.8	— 1.6	+ 7.9	+ 6.5	— 4.0	—	— 1.0	1282
Rousseau et al., 1972	10	— 2.3	— 9.2*	+ 7.5*	— 1.6	— 1.7	+ 1.6	— 4.7	630
	11	— 1.2	— 9.4*	+ 10.7	— 1.2	— 1.2	— 1.2	— 2.6	1063
	8	— 1.1	— 8.7*	+ 6.4	— 2.0	+ 1.9	— 1.0	— 4.0	1390

* = $P < 0.0.5$ ** = Mean of the $\dot{V}_{O_2}$ measured before and after physical training.

Abbreviations : HR = Heart Rate ;   Qs = Stroke Volume ;   Q = Cardiac Output ; $\dot{V}$ = Ventilation.

level of submaximal exercise while the cardiac output at a higher submaximal exercise was not modified. One is therefore faced with coronary patients to discrepancies similar to those observed in healthy subjects. With the exception of the patients of Frick et al. (1971) who were studied in supine posture, all other mentioned studies refer to upright exercise data. There are no other major differences between the experimental protocol of the studies presented in table 17 to account for the discrepancies between the results obtained, except perhaps for different belays between the moycardial infarction and the onset of training.

The studies of Detry et al. (1971) and Rousseau et al., (1972b) were conducted according to exactly the same common protocol with, however, one difference which might be of importance; all patients studied by Rousseau et al., (1972b) had their pre-training hemodynamic study 2 months after a well documented myocardial infarction requiring hospitalization, while in the other study the mean delay between the myocardial infarction and the beginning of the physical training program was 13 months. Interestingly, in their control group (table 17), Rousseau et al. (1972b) also found a significant increase in stroke volume, which confirms previous data by Frick et al. (1971). One may therefore question whether or not part of the results of Rousseau et al. (1972b) do not simply represent the spontaneous evolution of the stroke volume during the first few months after an acute myocardial infarction ; this tentative explanation could also contribute to explain the increased stroke volume reported by Frick and Katila (1968) and Frick et al., (1971) since all their patients were included in the training program 2 to 4 months after an acute myocardial infarction. The interval between the acute myocardial infarction and the onset of the training program was, however, much longer in the studies of Clausen et al. (1969) and Clausen and Trap-Jensen (1970) who reported variable effects of training on stroke volume. Further long-term hemodynamic studies on the effects of physical training after acute myocardial infarction, with double-blind repartition of the patients into a training and a control group, are needed to elucidate this problem.

In the comparison of the data presented in table 17, one essential element is unfortunately lacking, however, namely coronary arteriographic data ; it is indeed possible that differences in the anatomic state of the coronary arteries account partly for the different results.

3. Distribution of cardiac output.

The distribution of the submaximal cardiac output is also affected by physical training in coronary patients. Clausen and Trap-Jensen (1970) have indeed demonstrated that at a given level of submaximal exercise, the estimated splanchnic blood flow was higher after physical training ; this finding may be related to the lower relative severity of the exercise after physical conditioning (Rowell et al., 1964a). Higher splanchnic blood flow at submaximal exercise after training must be compensated by a decrease in one other regional flow ; the submaximal muscle blood flow (per 100 g of muscle) is indeed decreased after training of coronary patients (Clausen and Trap-Jensen, 1970). After training, the working muscles therefore have to extract a similar amount of oxygen from a lower muscle blood flow ; the latter is still further decreased when the total submaximal cardiac output is reduced after conditioning. Accordingly, the oxygen extraction capacity of the muscles is probably increased after physical training ; as in healthy sujects, this adaptation is probably based on an increased enzymatic activity of the skeletal muscles. These modifications in the working muscles could also account for the lower blood levels of lactic acid at submaximal exercise after training in coronary patients (Varnauskas et al., 1966, Bergman and Varnauskas, 1971).

C. Physical work capacity.

Many authors have indicated that physical training increased the physical work capacity of coronary patients but only a few studies include data measured at the maximal exercise level (Kash and Boyer, 1969; Detry et al., 1971 ; Detry and Bruce, 1971b ; Epstein et al., 1971).

Table 18 presents the results of a 3-month physical training program followed by 22 patients, 11 of

TABLE 18

Effects of physical training on the physical work capacity of coronary patients (from Detry and Bruce, 1971b, and Detry et al., 1971).

Number of patients	Age years	Parameter	Before training	After training	% change	P**
Angina pectoris 11	50.6	$\dot{V}_{O_2,SL}$ * HR max	18.7 130	24.7 143	+ 32 + 10	< 0.001 < 0.005
No angina pectoris 11	49	$\dot{V}_{O_2,max}$ * HR max	25.7 165	29.8 169	+ 16 + 2.5	< 0.001 NS
All patients 22	49.8	$\dot{V}_{O_2,SL}$ or $\dot{V}_{O_2,max}$ * HR max	22.2 147	27.2 156	+ 22.5 + 6	< 0.001 < 0.001

* $\dot{V}_{O_2}$ expressed in ml/kg.min ** Paired T test.

whom had exertional angina pectoris before physical training. Patients without angina pectoris presented a 16 % increase in the $\dot{V}_{O2,max}$ after physical training with a small and non-significant increase in the maximal heart rate. Patients with angina pectoris who had a lower pretraining physical work capacity increased their $\dot{V}_{O2,SL}$ by 32 % with physical training while their maximal heart rate increased by 10 % ; also 2 of these 11 patients were no longer limited by exertional anginal pain after training. As in healthy subjects, the most important increases in physical work capacity with training are presented by those patients who had the lowest pretraining $\dot{V}_{O2,max}$ or $\dot{V}_{O2,SL}$ (fig. 15) ; 3 of these 22 patients did not show

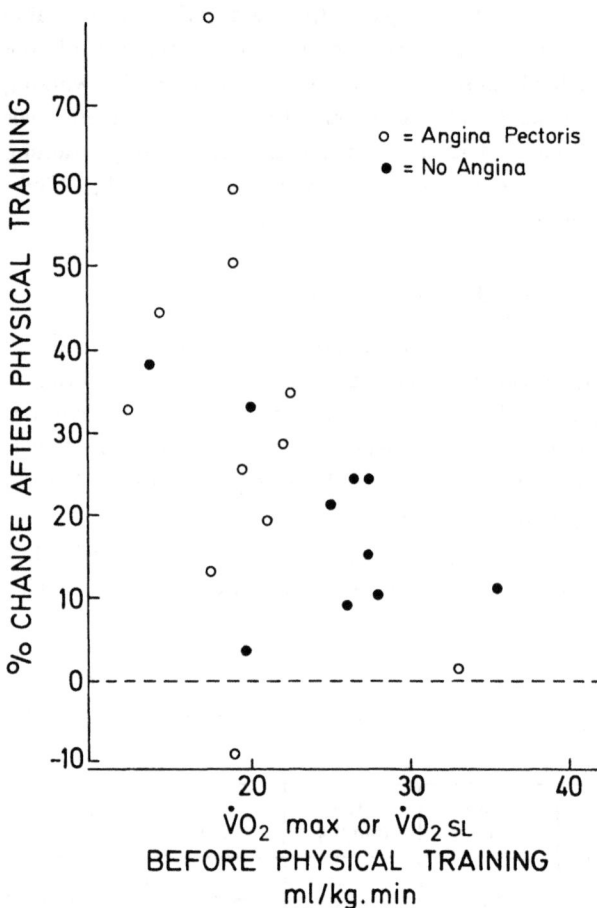

Fig. 15. — Percent change of $\dot{V}_{O2,max}$ and $\dot{V}_{O2,SL}$ after 3 months of physical training in relation to the absolute values measured before training in 22 patients. (from Detry and Bruce, 1971b, and Detry et al., 1971).

any improvement with physical training. When physical training is prolonged after the third month, there is still an 8.5 % increase in the physical work capacity from the third to the sixth month ($P < 0.05$; $n = 6$) ; further training from the seventh until the thirteenth

month causes only a small ($+ 4.5$ % ; $n = 12$) and non-significant increase in physical work capacity.

1. Patients without angina pactoris.

Increased physical work capacity of patients without angina pectoris is based on modifications of the hemo-dynamic determinants of the $\dot{V}_{O2,max}$ but no study includes hemodynamic data measured at the maximal exercise level. Calculated maximal cardiac output and maximal $a\text{-}v_{O2}$ difference before and after training (table 13) suggest that most of the increase in $\dot{V}_{O2,max}$ results from an expanded maximal $a\text{-}\bar{v}_{O2}$ difference (Detry et al., 1971) ; despite their limita-tions (see chapter 3) these calculated maximal values strongly suggest that physical training of coronary patients can lead to an increased $a\text{-}\bar{v}_{O2}$ difference at the maximal exercise level. Data of others also suggest that in some coronary patients, the increased $\dot{V}_{O2,max}$ results mostly from an increased cardiac output due to a greater stroke volume (Frick et al., 1968 ; Clausen et al., 1969 ; Rousseau et al., 1972b). But an accurate analysis of the factors responsible for the increased $\dot{V}_{O2,max}$ in patients with healed myocardial infarction requires hemodynamic data at the maximal exercise level.

2. Angina patients.

Increased $\dot{V}_{O2,SL}$ of angina patients after physical conditioning results essentially from the decreased heart rate, blood pressure and myocardial oxygen requirements during exercise ; the workload precipi-tating the anginal pain before training is indeed performed after training with lower myocardial oxygen requirements and the anginal pain is therefore prevented at this level of exercise. It is clearly de-monstrated, however, that after physical conditioning, the anginal pain occurs at significantly greater values of the pressure-rate product (Detry et al., 1971 ; Detry and Bruce, 1971b), triple product (Epstein et al., 1971) or tension-time index (Trap-Jensen and Clausen, 1971). These data suggest that after physical training, angina patients are able to meet greater myocardial oxygen requirements, i.e. the anginal threshold is higher ; these findings are difficult to interpret, however, since the electrocardiographic data after physical training (see chapter 2) do not suggest an improved oxygen supply to the myocardium (Detry and Bruce, 1971b ; 1971c). Psychological changes induced by physical training could also play a role by modifying the threshold of pain perception (Hellerstein, 1968).

D. Unsolved questions.

The improvement of many coronary patients with physical training is now well documented but, as already pointed out, the mechanisms of action of training are not yet well understood. The effects of training on heart volume and myocardial contractility at rest and during exercise should be measured since these parameters are important determinants of the myocardial oxygen requirements. Hopefully, hemodynamic studies at the maximal exercise level in patients with healed myocardial infarction will increase our understanding of these mechanisms but, from the data already collected, one may guess that, as in healthy subjects, physical training operates through several mechanisms in coronary patients.

One of the potential mechanisms of action of physical training in coronary patients is the development of a collateral coronary circulation. Research studies on animals have given contradictory results on this point (Eckstein, 1957; Kaplinsky et al., 1968) and it would be hazardous to extrapolate to humans data collected in animals with artificially created coronary heart disease. Coronarographic studies together with coronary blood flow determinations and studies of the myocardial metabolism will perhaps clarify this problem.

The effects of physical training on the long-term prognosis of coronary heart disease have still to be precised. The short-term prognosis of coronary heart disease is not worsened by training and some suggest an improvement of this prognosis (Gottheiner, 1969 ; Rechnitzer et al., 1972); it should be determined whether this improved prognosis results from physical activity by itself or rather from a better associated medical management with correction of risk factors such as hypertension, hyperlipidemia or obesity. Il will also be essential to define the relative advantages of physical training and myocardial revascularization surgery in order to better establish the therapeutical indications. The preventive effects of physical activity on the development of coronary heart disease in healthy subjects or in subjects with one or more risk factors are still being discussed (Fox and Paul, 1969); on current evidence, the existence of such a preventive action of physical activity cannot yet be positively affirmed and further research is needed (Keys, 1970b).

Other effects of physical training which do not have been discussed here, such as the effects of physical activity on the blood lipids, on the catecholamines metabolism and on the coagulation mechanisms, also raise many questions. In addition, the effects of training on the psychology of the patients and on their social and professional rehabilitation have to be defined ; the first studies on the economic aspect of the rehabilitation of cardiac patients indicate that it is a worthwhile effort (Helander, 1971).

CONCLUSIONS

Exercise testing is a very useful procedure in the evaluation of coronary patients and it should be considered as the most logical extension of the medical history and clinical examination of patients with documented or suspected coronary heart disease. Since coronary arteriography cannot be considered, for obvious reasons, as a routine diagnostic procedure, exercise electrocardiography has an essential role in the diagnosis of coronary artery disease ; objective evaluation of this diagnostic method reveals that it has a good sensitivity and an acceptable specificity.

Many questions remain unanswered, however. Clinical and epidemiological data indicate that the horizontal ST segment depression during or after exercise is the most reliable criterion for coronary insufficiency, but the mechanisms directly causing the depression of the ST segment remain largely unknown ; although hemodynamic and metabolic correlative studies confirm that this electrocardiographic pattern is related to an imbalance between myocardial oxygen needs and supply, the precise cause, metabolic or other, has still to be established. In addition the mechanisms responsible for the postexertional electrocardiographic pattern in coronary heart disease have still to be elucidated. The exact significance of the exertional electrocardiographic data collected in hypertensive patients or in patients with rheumatic valvular heart disease is still debated ; in this field, anatomo-electrocardiographical studies are obviously needed. The clinical meaning of the so-called « non specific » electrocardiographic findings should be determined from both correlative studies with arteriographic data and particularly from longitudinal studies which should define the long term prognosis of such abnormalities. Studies on exercise electrocardiography are still limited by the present difficulty to estimate easily and accurately the role played by factors such as the heart volume and the myocardial contractility. New investigation methods, mostly non-bleeding, should allow the role of these parameters to be determined.

Exercise testing is also the only way to estimate accurately the functional capacity of coronary patients, which can otherwise be grossly misinterpreted ; in this regard, testing up to the maximal exercise level appears to be the best method and its risks do not seem greater than those of submaximal exercise testing. Maximal exercise testing gives valuable information for the treatment and the rehabilitation of the patients and it also provides an objective baseline for the evaluation of the effects of a therapy. The factors limiting the $\dot{V}_{O_2,max}$ of patients with healed myocardial infarction (no angina pectoris) are not yet exactly defined. Data collected during submaximal exercise indicate that coronary patients have a lower stroke volume than healthy controls and also suggest that these patients cannot keep constant values of stroke volume when the severity of the exercise is increased. Hemodynamic studies at the maximal exercise level should precise the importance of this fall in the stroke volume at high exercise levels, and indicate whether or not coronary patients are also limited by peripheral factors ; studies of this kind combined with experimental assay of drugs or long-term therapy such as physical training will greatly develop our knoweledge of the pathophysiology of coronary heart disease.

The pathophysiology of exertional angina pectoris has been the subject of much research in recent years and the role of hemodynamic factors in the determination of the angina threshold is now well established ; since the oxygen consumption measured at the angina threshold does not fulfill the criteria for $\dot{V}_{O_2,max}$, it should be designated as sympton limited oxygen consumption ($\dot{V}_{O_2,SL}$). The substances or the mechanisms directly causing the anginal pain have still to be identified, however, and current evidence suggest that angina pectoris with exercise and ischemic ST changes are not determined by identical factors. Among the drugs used in the treatment of angina pectoris, nitroglycerin and beta-blocking agents appear to be the most powerful ; although the hemodynamic effects of these drugs have been extensively studied, their action on the coronary blood flow and its distribution have still to be determined in coronary patients.

Physical training of coronary patients constitutes a valuable therapeutic progress but its mechanisms of action have still to be better defined. Conflicting results in the literature probably indicate that physical training acts through several mechanisms ; long-term studies might however indicate that the discrepancies are more appearent than real since they could result from differences in the selection of the patients and/or various intervals between acute myocardial infarction and the onset of training. The possible effects of training on the coronary collateral circulation, on the total or regional coronary blood flow and on the myocardial metabolism have not yet been elucidated and future research studies on coronary patients should not overlook this aspect. In addition, the respective benefits and so the respective indications of exercise training and of myocardial revascularization surgery should be determined. The effects of physical activity on the primary and secondary prevention of coronary heart disease are now being extensively studied and the results are still controversial ; in this situation, however, it seems most logical to advise physical activity since it has other well demonstrated valuable effects.

CONCLUSIONS

Les tests d'efforts occupent une place importante dans le diagnostic de l'insuffisance coronarienne ainsi que dans l'évaluation fonctionnelle des malades coronariens ; l'effort physique, effectué sous surveillance médicale, représenté également un des aspects du traitement de la maladie coronarienne stabilisée.

L'électrocardiographie d'effort constitue une méthode de diagnostic à la fois sensible et spécifique ainsi qu'en témoignent les pourcentages peu élevés de diagnostics faussement négatifs ou faussement positifs ; à cet égard la supériorité des tests d'efforts maximaux est bien établie et leur risque ne paraît pas plus grand que celui des tests d'efforts sous-maximaux. De nombreux problèmes restent toutefois en suspens. Alors que les études cliniques et épidémiologiques ont démontré qu'une dépression horizontale du segment ST pendant ou après l'effort constituait un critère fidèle d'insuffisance coronarienne, les mécanismes responsables de cette anomalie électrocardiographique sont mal connus ; des travaux basés sur l'adaptation hémodynamique et métabolique à l'effort ont confirmé que la dépression du segment ST et son importance reflétait un déséquilibre entre les besoins en oxygène du myocarde et l'apport d'oxygène au myocarde, mais les facteurs directement responsables au niveau cellulaire doivent encore être précisés. Les tracés enregistrés après l'effort ont souvent un aspect différent de ceux enregistrés pendant l'effort mais les raisons de cette différence ne sont pas claires. L'interprétation des tracés électrocardiographiques enregistrés à l'effort chez des malades hypertendus ou valvulaires reste délicate ; seules des études confrontant des données anatomiques et électrocardiographiques permettront de préciser la valeur de l'électrocardiogramme d'effort chez ces malades. Les anomalies dites aspécifiques de la repolarisation posent également des problèmes d'interprétation car le devenir à long terme des patients présentant ces anomalies n'est pas bien connu. Les études électrocardiographiques restent toutefois limitées par la difficulté d'estimer actuellement le rôle exact joué par des facteurs comme la contractilité myocardique ou le volume ventriculaire gauche.

Les tests d'efforts constituent aussi la seule méthode de mesure de la capacité physique des coronariens ; les données recueillies au repos ne permettent en effet qu'une estimation assez grossière de la capacité physique de ces patients. Dans ce sens, les tests d'efforts maximaux représentent certainement l'approche la plus objective et ils fournissent des données extrêmement utiles pour le traitement et la réadaptation des malades coronariens ; ils permettent en outre d'apprécier objectivement les résultats d'un traitement qu'il soit médical ou chirurgical. Les facteurs qui limitent la capacité physique (ou consommation maximale d'oxygène - $V_{O2,max}$) des malades coronariens sans angor d'effort restent à préciser car à notre connaissance, les paramètres hémodynamiques au cours de l'effort maximal n'ont pas encore été mesurés chez ces malades. Les résultats obtenus lors de l'effort sous-maximal démontrent que le débit systolique des coronariens est plus bas que celui des sujets sains ; il semble, en outre, que contrairement aux sujets normaux, les coronariens présentent une baisse progressive du débit systolique lorsque l'intensité relative de l'effort s'accroît. Les recherches futures devront préciser l'importance réelle de cette chute du débit systolique lors de l'effort maximal et définir ainsi le rôle exact joué par les facteurs périphériques dans la limitation fonctionnelle des coronariens sans angor.

Ces dernières années, la physiopathologie de l'angine de poitrine d'effort a fait l'objet de nombreux travaux qui ont mis en évidence l'importance des facteurs hémodynamiques dans le déclenchement de l'angor d'effort et ont ainsi permis l'introduction de la notion de seuil angineux. Etant donné que la consommation d'oxygène mesurée au moment de l'apparition de la douleur angineuse ne répond pas aux critères définissant la consommation maximale d'oxygène, le terme de consommation d'oxygène limitée par les symptômes ($\dot{V}_{O2,SL}$) parait préférable. Bien que l'angine de poitrine d'effort soit l'un des symptômes les plus caractéristique d'ischémie myocardique, les mécanismes ou les facteurs directement responsables de l'apparition de la douleur n'ont pas encore été identifiés ; il semble toutefois établi que le déclenchement de la douleur angineuse et l'apparition ou l'importance des modifications électrocardiographiques ne sont pas contrôlés par des facteurs identiques. Parmi les drogues utilisées dans le traitement et la prévention de l'angine de poitrine d'effort, les dérivés nitrés et les agents bêta-bloquants occupent une place toute particulière, du fait de leur action très puissante ; ces drogues ont fait l'objet de nombreux travaux hémodynamiques mais leurs effets éventuels sur le débit coronaire et sa distribution n'ont pas encore été mesurés chez les coronariens.

L'utilité de l'entraînement physique dans le traitement et la réadaptation des malades coronariens est bien établie ; ses effets bénéfiques résultent essentiellement d'une diminution de la fréquence cardiaque et de la pression artérielle à l'effort sous-maximal. Les effets de l'entraînement physique sur le débit systolique et le débit cardiaque restent toutefois controversés ; il est possible que les résultats divergents de la littérature soient dus à des différences dans la sélection des malades et à des délais variables entre l'infarctus myocardique et le début de la réadaptation physique. L'action de l'entraînement physique sur la circulation coronarienne collatérale ainsi que sur le débit coronarien total ou régional n'a pas encore été établie. Des travaux de recherche devront également déterminer les résultats comparatifs de l'entraînement physique et de la chirurgie de revascularisation myocardique, ceci dans le but de mieux poser les indications thérapeutiques. Le rôle de l'activité physique dans la prévention primaire et secondaire de la maladie coronarienne est maintenant l'objet de nombreuses études qui n'ont pas encore apporté d'éléments décisifs en faveur d'une telle action préventive ; l'entraînement physique a toutefois d'autres effets favorables bien démontrés qui justifient largement sont utilisation dans le traitement de la maladie coronarienne.

BIBLIOGRAPHY

ABLAD B. : A study of the mechanisms of the hemodynamic effects of hydralazine in man. — *Acta Pharmacol.*, **20** : 1-53, 1963.

ANDREW G.M., GUZMAN C.A., BECKLAKE M.R. : Effect of athletic training on exercise cardiac output. — *J. appl. Physiol.*, **21** : 603-608, 1966.

ARBORELIUS M. Jr., LECEROF H., MALM A., MALMBORG R.O. : Acute effect of nitroglycerin on haemodynamic of angina pectoris. — *Brit. Heart J.*, **30** : 407-411, 1968.

ARESKOG N.H., ADOLFSSON L. : Effects of a cardioselective beta-adrenergic blocker (ICI 50172) at exercise in angina pectoris. — *Brit. med. J.*, **2** : 601-603, 1969.

ARONOW W.S., DENDINGER J., ROKAW S.N. : Heart rate and carbon monoxide level after smoking high-, low-, and non-nicotine cigarettes. A study in male patients with angina pectoris. — *Ann. Int. Med.*, **74** : 697-702, 1971b.

ARONOW W.S., PAPAGEORGE'S N.P., UYEAMA R.R., CASSIDY J. : Maximal treadmill stress test correlated with post-exercise phonocardiogram in normal subjects. — *Circulation*, **43** : 884-888, 1971a.

ARONOW W.S., ROKAW S.N. : Carboxyhemoglobin caused by smoking nonnicotine cigarettes. Effects in angina pectoris. — *Circulation*, **44** : 782-788, 1971.

ARONOW W.S., UYEYAMA R.R., CASSIDY J., NEBOLON J. : Resting and postexercise phonocardiogram and electrocardiogram in patients with angina pectoris and in normal subjects. — *Circulation*, **43** : 273-277, 1971c.

ÅSTRAND I. : Aerobic work capacity in men and women with special reference to age. — *Acta physiol. scand.*, **49**, suppl. 169, 1960, 92 p.

ÅSTRAND I. : Electrocardiographic changes in relation to the type of exercise, the work load, age and sex, p. 309-322 in BLACKBURN H. : Measurements in exercise electrocardiography. C.C. Thomas, Springfield, 1969, 488 p.

ÅSTRAND P.O., CUDDY T.E., SALTIN B., STENBERG J. : Cardiac output during submaximal and maximal work. — *J. appl. Physiol.*, **19** : 268-274, 1964.

ÅSTRAND I., LUNDMAN T. : The exercise electrocardiogram in coronary heart disease. Its prognostic value. — *Scand. J. clin. Lab. Invest.*, **22** : 301-306, 1968.

ÅSTRAND P.O. : Experimental studies of physical working capacity in relation to sex and age. Munksgaard, Copenhagen, 1952, 71 p.

ÅSTRAND P.O., EKBLOM B., MESSIN R., SALTIN B., STENBERG J. : Intra-arterial blood pressure during exercise with different muscle groups. — *J. appl. Physiol.*, **20** : 253-256, 1965.

ÅSTRAND P.O. ENGSTRÖM L., ERIKSSON B., KARLBERG P., NYLANDER I., SALTIN B., THOREN C. Girl swimmers. — *Acta Paediat.*, **52**, suppl. 147, 1963.

ÅSTRAND P.O., RODAHL K.R. : Textbook of work physiology, McGraw-Hill Book Cy, New York, 1970, 669 p.

ÅSTRAND P.O., RYHMING I. : A nomogram for calculation of aerobic capacity (physical fitness) from pulse rate during submaximal work. — *J. appl. Physiol.*, **7** : 218-221, 1954.

ÅSTRAND P.O., SALTIN B. : Oxygen uptake during the first minutes of heavy muscular exercise. — *J. appl. Physiol.*, **16** : 971-976, 1961a.

ÅSTRAND P.O., SALTIN B. : Maximal oxygen uptake and heart rate in various types of muscular activity. — *J. appl. Physiol.*, **16** : 977-981, 1961b.

ATTERHÖG J.H., EKELUND L.G., KAIJSER L. : Electrocardiographic abnormalities during exercise 3 weeks to 18 months after anterior myocardial infarction. — *Brit. Heart J.*, **33** : 871-877, 1971.

BALCON R., HOY J., MALLOY W., SOWTON E. : Haemodynamic comparisons of atrial pacing and exercise in patients with angina pectoris. — *Brit. Heart J.*, **31** : 168-171, 1969.

BARRY A.J., DALY J.W., PRUETT E.D.R., STEINMETZ J.R., BIRKHEAD N.C., RODAHL K. : Effects of physical training in patients who have had myocardial infarction. — *Amer. J. Cardiol.*, **17** : 1-8, 1966.

BATTOCK D.J., ALVAREZ H., CHIDSEY C.A. : Effects of propranolol and isosorbide dinitrate on exercise performance and adrenergic activity in patients with angina pectoris. — *Circulation*, **39** : 157-169, 1969.

BECKER L.C., FORTUIN N.J., PITT B. : Effect of ischemia and antianginal drugs on the distribution of radioactive microspheres in the canine left ventricle. — *Circulat. Res.*, **28** : 263-269, 1971.

BELLET S., ELIAKIM M., DELILYANNIS S., LA VAN D. : Radioelectrocardiography during exercise in patients with angina pectoris. Comparison with the postexercise electrocardiogram. — *Circulation*, **25** : 5-14, 1962.

BELLET S., MULLER O.F., LA VAN D., NICHOLS G.J., HERRING A.B. : Radioelectrocardiography during exercise in patients with the anginal syndrome. Use of multiple leads. — *Circulation*, **29** : 366-375, 1964.

BELLET S., ROMAN L. : Comparison of the double two-step test and the maximal exercise treadmill test. Studies in coronary prone subjects. — *Circulation*, **36** : 238-244, 1967.

BELLET S., ROMAN L.R., NICHOLS G.J., MULLER O.F. : Detection of coronary prone subjects in a normal population by radioelectrocardiographic exercise test. Follow-up studies. — *Amer. J. Cardiol.*, **19** : 783-787, 1967.

BENESTAD A.M. : Determination of physical work capacity and exercise tolerance in cardiac patients. — *Acta med. scand.*, 183 : 521-529, 1968.

BERGMAN H., VARNAUSKAS E. : The hemodynamic effects of physical training in coronary patients. — *Med. Sport*, 4 : 138-147, 1970.

BERNE R.M. : Regulation of coronary blood flow. — *Physiol. Rev.*, 44 : 1-29, 1964.

BERNE R.M., DE GEEST H., LEVY M.N. : Influence of the cardiac nerves on coronary resistance. — *Amer. J. Physiol.*, 203 : 763-769, 1965.

BERNE R.M., LEVY M.N. : Cardiovascular physiology. C.V. Mosby Cy, Saint Louis, 1967, 254 p.

BERNSTEIN L., FRIESINGER G.C., LICHTLEN P.R., ROSS R.S.: The effect of nitroglycerin on the systemic and coronary circulation in man and dogs. Myocardial blood flow measured with Xenon^{133}. — *Circulation*, 33: 107-116, 1966.

BEVEGÅRD S., FREYSCHUSS U., STRANDELL T. : Circulatory adaptation to arm and leg exercise in supine and sitting position. — *J. appl. Physiol.*, 21 : 37-46, 1966.

BEVEGÅRD S., HOLMGREN A., JONSSON B. : The effect of body position on the circulation at rest and during exercise, with special reference to the influence on the stroke volume. — *Acta physiol. scand.*, 49 : 279-298, 1960.

BEVEGÅRD S., HOLMGREN A., JONSSON B. : Circulatory studies in well trained athletes at rest and during heavy exercise, with special reference to stroke volume and the influence of body position. — *Acta physiol. scand.*, 57 : 26-50, 1963.

BEVEGÅRD S., SHEPHERD J.T. : Changes in tome of limb veins during supine exercise. — *J. appl. Physiol.*, 20 : 1-8, 1965.

BEVEGÅRD S., SHEPHERD J.T. : Reaction in man of resistance and capacity vessels in forearm and hand to leg exercise. — *J. appl. Physiol.*, 21 : 123-132, 1966a.

BEVEGÅRD S., SHEPHERD J.T. : Circulatory effects of stimulating the carotid arterial stretch receptors in man at rest and during exercise. — *J. clin. Invest.*, 45 : 132-142, 1966b.

BEVEGÅRD S., SHEPHERD J.T. : Regulation of the circulation during exercise in man. — *Physiol. Rev.*, 47 : 178-213, 1967.

BING R.J., BENNISH A., BLUEMCHEN G., COHEN A., GALLAGHER J.P., ZALESKI E.J. : The determination of coronary flow equivalent with coincidence counting technic. — *Circulation*, 29 : 833-846, 1964.

BJÖRNTROP P., FAHLEN M., HOLM J., SCHERSTEN T., STENBERG J. : Changes in the activity of skeletal muscle succinic oxydase after training, p. 138-142 in LARSON O.A., MALMBORG R.O. : Coronary disease and physical fitness, Munksgaard, Copenhagen, 1971, 277 p.

BLACKBURN H. : Measurement in exercise electrocardiography. C.C. Thomas, Springfield, 1969, 488 p.

BLACKBURN H. : The exercise electrocardiogram. Technological, procedural and conceptual developments, p. 220-258 in BLACKBURN H. : Measurements in exercise electrocardiography, C.C. Thomas, Springfield, 1969, 488 p.

BLACKBURN H., KATIGBAK R. : What electrocardiographic leads to take after exercise ? — *Amer. Heart J.*, 67 : 184-185, 1964.

BLACKBURN H., TAYLOR H.L., KEYS A. : Coronary heart disease in seven countries. 16. The electrocardiogram in prediction of five-years coronary heart disease incidence among men aged forty through fifty-nine. — *Circulation*, 41, suppl. 1 : 154-161, 1970.

BLACKBURN H., TAYLOR H.L., OKAMOTO N., RAUTAHARJU P., MITCHELL P.L., KERKHOF A.C. : Standardization of the exercise electrocardiogram. A systematic comparison of chest lead configurations employed for monitoring during exercise, p. 101-133 in KARVONEN M.J., BARRY A. : Physical activity and the heart, C.C. Thomas, Springfield, 1966, 405 p.

BLACKBURN H. and a TECHNICAL GROUP : The exercise electrocardiogram : differences in interpretation. Report of a technical group on exercise electrocardiography. — *Amer. J. Cardiol.*, 21 : 871-880, 1968.

BLACKMON J.R., ROWELL L.B., KENNEDY J.W., TWISS R.D., CONN R.D. : Physiological significance of maximal oxygen intake in « pure » mitral stenosis. — *Circulation*, 36 : 497-510, 1967.

BLOMQVIST G. : The Frank lead exercise electrocardiogram. A quantitative study based on averaging technic and digital computer analysis. — *Acta med. scand.*, 178, suppl. 440, 1965, 98 p.

BLOMQVIST G. : Use of exercise testing for diagnostic and functional evaluation of patients with arteriosclerotic heart disease. — *Circulation*, 44 : 1120-1136, 1971.

BLOOMER W.E., ELLESTAD M.H., BELAND A.J., COPE J.A., PALAREA E.R. : Evaluation of myocardial revascularization with arterial implants. An objective study using electrocardiography and maximal stress testing. — *Ann. int. Med.*, 73 : 913-919, 1970.

BOERTH R.C., COVELL J.W., POOL P.E., ROSS J. : Increased myocardial oxygen consumption and contractile state associated with increased heart rate in dogs. — *Circulat. Res.*, 24 : 725-734, 1969.

BONJER F.H. : Physical working capacity and energy expenditure, p. 23-30 in DENOLIN et al : Ergometry in Cardiology, Boehringer, Mannheim, 1968, 252 p.

BOTTIN R., PETIT J.M., DEROANNE R., PIRNAY F., JUCHMES J. : Mesures comparées de la consommation maximum d'O_2 par paliers de 1 ou 2 minutes. — *Int. Z. angew. Physiol.*, 29 : 11-17, 1970.

BRAUNWALD E. : Control of myocardial oxygen consumption. Physiologic and clinical considerations. — *Amer. J. Cardiol.*, 27 : 416-432, 1971.

BRAUNWALD E., SONNENBLICK E.H., ROSS J., GLICK G., EPSTEIN S.E. : An analysis of the cardiac response to exercise. — *Circulat. Res.*, 22, suppl. 1 : 44-58, 1967a.

BRAUNWALD E., EPSTEIN S.E., GLICK G., WECHSLER A.S., BRAUNWALD N.S. : Relief of angina pectoris by electrical stimulation of the carotid-sinus nerves. — *N. Engl. J. Med.*, 277 : 1278-1283, 1967b.

BRODY A.J. : Master two-step test in clinically unselected patients. — *J. Amer. med. Ass.*, 171 : 1195-1198, 1959.

BROUHA L., SMITH P.E., DE LANNE R., MAXFIELD M.E. : Physiological reactions of men and women during muscular activity and recovery in various environments. — *J. appl. Physiol.*, 16 : 133-140, 1960.

BROUWERS J., PATIGNY J., LAVENNE F. : Critères de sélection pour le travail à hautes températures. — *Rev. Inst. Hyg. Mines*, 23 : 139-149, 1968.

BRUCE R.A. : Manual of exercise testing. University of Washington, Seattle, 1970, 50 p.

BRUCE R.A. : Exercise testing of patients with coronary heart disease. Principles and standards for evaluation. — *Ann. Clin. Res.*, 3 : 323-332, 1971.

BRUCE R.A., BLACKMON J.R., JONES J.W., STRAIT G. : Exercise testing in adult normal subjects and cardiac patients. — *Pediatrics*, 32 : 742-756, 1963.

BRUCE R.A., HORNSTEN T.R. : Exercise stress testing in evaluation of patients with ischemic heart disease. — *Progr. cardiovasc. Dis.*, 11 : 371-390, 1969.

BRUCE R.A., HORNSTEN T.R., BLACKMON J.R. : Myocardial infarction after normal responses to maximal exercise. — *Circulation*, 38 : 552-558, 1968.

BRUCE R.A., KLUGE A. : Defibrillatory treatment of exertional cardiac arrest in seven coronary patients. — *J. Amer. med. Ass.*, 216 : 653-658, 1971.

BRUCE R.A., MAZZARELLA J.A., JORDAN J.W., GREEN E. : Quantification of QRS and ST segment responses to exercise. — *Amer. Heart J.*, 71 : 455-466, 1966.

BRUCE R.A., ROWELL L.B., BLACKMON J.R., DOAN A. : Cardiovascular function tests. — *Heart Bull.*, 14 : 9-16, 1965.

BURKART F., BAROLD S., SOWTON E. : Hemodynamic effects of repeated exercise. — *Amer. J. Cardiol.*, 20 : 509-515, 1967.

BUSKIRK E., TAYLOR L.T. : Maximal oxygen intake and its relation to body composition with special reference to chronic physical activity and obesity. — *J. appl. Physiol.*, 11 : 72-78, 1957.

CASE R.B., NASSER M.G., CRAMPTON R.S. : Biochemical aspects of early myocardial ischemia. — *Amer. J. Cardiol.*, 24 : 766-775, 1969.

CASE R.B., ROSELLE H.A., CRAMPTON R.S. : Relation of ST depression to metabolic and hemodynamic events. — *Cardiologia*, 48 : 32-41, 1966.

CASTENFORS J., PISCATOR M. : Renal hemodynamics, urine flow and urinary protein excretion during exercise in supine position at different loads. — *Acta med. scand.*, 472 : 231-244, 1967.

CHAMBERLAIN D.A. : Effects of beta adrenergic blockade on heart size. — *Amer. J. Cardiol.*, 18 : 321-328, 1966.

CHAPMAN C.B., FISHER J.N., SPROULE B.J. : Behavior of stroke volume at rest and during exercise in human beings. — *J. clin. Invest.*, 39 : 1208-1213, 1960.

CHAPMAN C.B., FRASER R.S. : Studies on the effect of exercise on cardiovascular function. III. Cardiovascular response to exercise in patients with healed myocardial infarction. — *Circulation*, 9 : 347-351, 1954.

CHIANG B., ALEXANDER E.R., BRUCE R.A., THOMPSON D.J., TING N. : Factors related to ST segment depression after exercie in middle-age chinese men. — *Circulation*, 40 : 315-325, 1969.

CLAUSEN J.P., LARSEN O.A., TRAP-JENSEN J. : Physical training in the management of coronary artery disease. — *Circulation*, 40 : 143-154, 1969.

CLAUSEN J.P., TRAP-JENSEN J. : Effects of training on the distribution of cardiac output in patients with coronary heart disease. — *Circulation*, 42 : 611-624, 1970.

CLAUSEN J.P., TRAP-JENSEN J., LASSEN N.A. : The effects of training on the heart rate during arm and leg exercise. — *Scand. J. clin. Lab. Invest.*, 26 : 295-301, 1970.

COBB L.A., JOHNSON W.P. : Hemodynamic relationships of anaerobic metabolism and plasma free fatty acids during prolonged, strenuous exercise in trained and untrained subjects. — *J. clin. Invest.*, 42 : 800-810, 1963.

COHEN L.S., ELLIOTT W.C., ROLETT E.L., GORLIN R. : Hemodynamic studies during angina pectoris. — *Circulation*, 31 : 409-416, 1965.

COHN P.F., VOKONAS P.S., HERMAN M.V., GORLIN R. : Postexercise electrocardiogram in patients with abnormal resting electrocardiogram. — *Circulation*, 43 : 648-654, 1971.

COLEMAN H.N., SONNENBLICK E.H., BRAUNWALD E : Myocardial oxygen consumption associated with external work. The Fenn effect. — *Amer. J. Physiol.*, 217 : 291-296, 1969.

COVELL J.W., BRAUNWALD E., ROSS J., SONNENBLICK E.H. : Studies on digitalis. XVI. Effects on myocardial oxygen consumption. — *J. clin. Invest.*, 45 : 1535-1542, 1966.

DATEY K.K., MISRA S.N. : The evaluation of two-step exercise test in patients with heart disease of different etiologies. — *Dis. Chest.*, 53 : 294-300, 1968.

DAVIS F.W., SCARBOROUGH W.R., MASON R.E., SINGEWALD M.L., BAKER B.M. : The effects of exercise and smoking on the electrocardiogram and ballistocardiogram of normal subjects and patients with coronary artery disease. — *Amer. Heart J.,* 46 : 529-542, 1953.

DEMANY M.A., TAMBE A., ZIMMERMAN H.A. : Correlation between coronary arteriography and the post-exercise electrocardiogram. — *Amer. J. Cardiol.,* 19 : 526-530, 1967.

DENOLIN H., MESSIN R., DEGRE S., VANDERMOTEN P., DE COSTER A. : Adaptation cardio-circulatoire au cours de l'effort musculaire : aspects physiologiques et applications pratiques. — *Acta Cardiol.,* 21 : 663-709, 1966.

DETRY J-M. R., BRUCE R.A. : Effects of nitroglycerin on « maximal » oxygen intake and exercise electrocardiogram in coronary heart disease. — *Circulation,* 43 : 155-163, 1971a.

DETRY J-M. R., BRUCE R.A. : Effects of physical training on exertional ST segment depression in coronary heart disease. — *Circulation,* 44 : 390-396, 1971b.

DETRY J-M. R., BRUCE R.A. : Divergent effects of physical training and nitroglycerin in coronary heart disease. — *Ann. int. Med.,* 74 : 819, 1971c.

DETRY J-M. R., GERIN M.G., CHARLIER A.A., BRASSEUR L.A. : Hemodynamic and thermal aspects of prolonged intermittent exercise. — *Int. Z. angew. Physiol.,* 30 : 171-185, 1972a.

DETRY J-M. R., PIETTE F., BRASSEUR L.A. : Hemodynamic determinants of exercise ST segment depression in coronary patients. — *Circulation,* 42 : 593-599, 1970.

DETRY J.-M. R., ROUSSEAU M., VANDENBROUCKE G., KUSUMI F., BRASSEUR L.A., BRUCE R.A. : Increased arteriovenous oxygen difference after physical training in coronary heart disease. — *Circulation,* 44 : 109-118, 1971.

DETRY J.-M. R. : WYSS C., ROWELL L.B. : Increased forearm venous compliance during exercise with nitroglycerin. In preparation, 1972b.

DIEUDONNE J.M. : Tissue-cavitary difference pressure of dog left ventricle. — *Amer. J. Physiol.,* 213 : 101-106, 1967.

DOAN A.E., PETERSON D.R., BLACKMON J.R., BRUCE R.A. : Myocardial ischemia after maximal exercise in healthy men. A method for detecting potential coronary heart disease. — *Amer. Heart J.,* 69 : 11-21, 1965.

DOUGLAS F.G.V., BECKLAKE M.R. : Effect of seasonal training on maximal cardiac output. — *J. appl. Physiol.,* 25 : 600-605, 1968.

DOYLE J.T., KINCH S.H. : The prognosis of an abnormal electrocardiographic stress test. — *Circulation,* 41 : 545-555, 1970.

DUNLOP D., SHANKS R.G. : Selective blockade of adrenoceptive receptors in the heart. — *Brit. J. Pharmacol.,* 32 : 201-218, 1968.

DWYER E.M. : Left ventricular pressure-volume alterations and regional disorders of contraction during myocardial ischemia induced by atrial pacing. — *Circulation,* 42 : 1111-1122, 1970.

ECKSTEIN R.W. : Effect of exercise and coronary artery narrowing on coronary collateral circulation. — *Circulat. Res.,* 5 : 230-235, 1957.

EKBLOM B. : Effect of training on adolescent boys. — *J. appl. Physiol.,* 27 : 350-355, 1969.

EKBLOM B., ÅSTRAND P.O., SALTIN B., STENBERG J., WALLSTRÖM B. : Effects of training on the circulatory response to exercise. — *J. appl. Physiol.,* 24 : 518-528, 1968.

EKBLOM B., HERMANSEN L. : Cardiac output in athletes. — *J. appl. Physiol.,* 25 : 619-625, 1968.

EKELUND L.G. : Circulatory and respiratory adaptation during prolonged exercise in the supine position. — *Acta physiol. scand.,* 68 : 382-396, 1966.

EKELUND L.G. : Circulatory and respiratory adaptation during prolonged exercise of moderate intensity in the sitting position. — *Acta physiol. scand.,* 69 : 327-340, 1967a.

EKELUND L.G. : Circulatory and respiratory adaptation during prolonged exercise. — *Acta physiol. scand.,* 70, suppl. 292, 1967b, 38 p.

EKELUND L.G., HOLMGREN A. : Circulatory and respiratory adaptation during long term, non steady state exercise, in the sitting position. — *Acta Physiol. Scand.,* 62 : 240-255, 1964.

EKMEKCI A., TOYOSHIMA H., KWOCZYNSKI J.K., NAGAYA T., PRINZMETAL M. : Angina pectoris. IV. Clinical and experimental difference between ischemia with S-T elevation and ischemia with S-T depression. — *Amer. J. Cardiol.,* 7 : 412-426, 1961.

ELIOT R.S., BRATT G. : The paradox of myocardial ischemia and necrosis in young women with normal coronary arteriograms. Relation to abnormal hemoglobin-oxygen dissociation. — *Amer. J. Cardiol.,* 23 : 633-638, 1969.

ELLESTAD M.H., ALLEN W., WAN M.C.K., KEMP G.L. : Maximal treadmill stress testing for cardiovascular evaluation. — *Circulation,* 39 : 517-522, 1969.

EPSTEIN S.E., REDWOOD D.R., GOLDSTEIN R.E., BEISER G.D., ROSING D.R., GLANCY D.L., REIS R.L., STINSON E.B. : Angina pectoris : pathophysiology, evaluation and treatment. — *Ann. int. Med.,* 75 : 263-296, 1971.

EPSTEIN S.E., ROBINSON B.F., KAHLER R.L., BRAUNWALD E. : Effects of beta-adrenergic blockade on the cardiac response to maximal and submaximal exercise in man. — *J. clin. Invest.,* 44 : 1745-1753, 1965.

EPSTEIN S.E., STAMPFER M., BEISER G.B. : Effects of a reduction in environmental temperature on the circulatory response to exercise in man. — *New Engl. J. Med.,* 280 : 7-11, 1969.

FALLS H.B. : The relative energy requirements of various physical activities in relation to physiological strain. — J.S.C. med. Ass., 65 : 8-11, 1969.

FEIGL E.O. : Parasympathetic control of coronary blood flow in dogs. — Circulat. Res., 25 : 509-519, 1969.

FITZGERALD J.G., SCALES B. : Effect of a new adrenergic beta-blocking agent (ICI 50172) on heart rate in relation to its blood levels. — Int. J. clin. Pharmacol., 1 : 467-474, 1958.

FOLIATH F. : Central venous pressure and cardiac output during exercise in coronary disease. — Brit. Heart J., 29 : 714-718, 1967.

FORD A.B., HELLERSTEIN H.K. : Energy cost of the Master two-step test. — J. Amer. med. Ass., 164 : 1868-1874, 1957.

FORTUIN N.J., FRIESINGER G.C. : Exercise-induced S-T segment elevation. Clinical, electrocardiographic and arteriographic studies in twelve patients. — Amer. J. Med., 49 : 459-464, 1970.

FOX S.M., PAUL O. : Physical activity and coronary heart disease. — Amer. J. Cardiol., 23 : 298-306, 1969.

FRETEUR J.P., FERNANDEZ H., COUPEZ J.M., BRASSEUR L.A. : Les anomalies non spécifiques de la repolarisation. A propos de 25 observations. — Rev. Inst. Hyg. Mines, 21 : 237-263, 1966.

FRETEUR J.P., GOENEN M., FERNANDEZ H., BRASSEUR L.A. : Les anomalies non spécifiques de la repolarisation ventriculaire. — Acta Cardiol., 25 : 119-143, 1970.

FRICK M.H., BALCON R., CROSS D., SOWTON E. : Hemodynamic effects of nitroglycerin in patients with angina pectoris studied by an atrial pacing method. — Circulation, 37 : 160-168, 1968.

FRICK M.H., KATILA M. : Hemodynamic consequences of physical training after myocardial infarction. — Circulation, 37 : 192-202, 1968.

FRICK M.H., KATILA M. : Cardio-selective beta-adrenergic inhibition by practolol in angina pectoris. — Ann. clin. Res., 2 : 96-101, 1970.

FRICK M.H., KATILA M., SJÖGREN A.L. : Cardiac function and physical training after myocardial infarction, p. 43-47 in LARSEN O.A., MALMBORG R.O. : Physical fitness and coronary heart disease, Munksgaard, Copenhagen, 1971, 277 p.

FRICK M.H., KONTTINEN A., SARAJAS H.S. : Effects of physical training on circulation at rest and during exercise. — Amer. J. Cardiol., 12 : 142-163, 1963.

FRIEDBERG C.K., JAFFE H.L., PORDY L., CHESKY K. : The two-step exercise electrocardiogram. A double blind evaluation of its use in the diagnostic of angina pectoris. — Circulation, 26 : 1254-1260, 1962.

FURBERG C. : Adrenergic beta-blockade and electrocardiographical ST-T changes. — Acta med. scand., 181 : 21-32, 1967.

FURBERG C. : Effects of beta-adrenergic blockade on ECG, physical working capacity and central circulation with special reference to autonomic imbalance. — Acta med. scand., 183, suppl. 488, 1968, 46 p.

GENSINI G.C., BRUTO da COSTA B.C. : The coronary collateral circulation in living man. — Amer. J. Cardiol., 24 : 393-400, 1969.

GIANELLY R.E., TREISTER B.L., HARRISSON D.C. : The effect of propranolol on exercise-induced ischemic ST segment depression. — Amer. J. Cardiol., 24 : 161-165, 1969.

GOENEN M., FERNANDEZ H., BRASSEUR L.A. : Intérêt des épreuves d'effort à charge croissante dans le diagnostic électrocardiographique de l'angine de poitrine. — Acta Cardiol., 25 : 1-28, 1970.

GOLDSTEIN R.E., REDWOOD D.R., ROSING D.R., BEISER G.D., EPSTEIN S.E. : Alterations in the circulatory response to exercise following a meal and their relationship to postprandial angina pectoris. — Circulation, 44 : 90-100, 1971b.

GOLDSTEIN R.E., ROSING D.R., REDWOOD D.R., BEISER G.D., EPSTEIN S.E. : Clinical and circulatory effects of isosorbide dinitrate. Comparison with nitroglycerin. — Circulation, 43 : 629-640, 1971a.

GOLLNICK P.D., KING D.W. : Effect of exercise and training on mitochondria of rat skeletal muscle. — Amer. J. Physiol., 216 : 1502-1509, 1969.

GOOCH A.S., McCONNEL D. : Analysis of transient arrythmias and conduction disturbances occuring during submaximal treadmill exercise. — Progr. cardiovasc. Dis., 13 : 293-307, 1970.

GORLIN R. : Regulation of coronary blood flow. — Brit. Heart J., 33 : 9-14, 1971.

GORLIN R., BRACHFELD N., MacLEOD C., BOPP P. : Effect of nitroglycerin on the coronary circulation in patients with coronary artery disease or increased left ventricular work. — Circulation, 19 : 705-718, 1959.

GORLIN R., KLEIN M.D., SULLIVAN J.M. : Prospective correlative study of ventricular aneurysm. Mechanistic concepts and clinical recognition. — Amer. J. Med., 42 : 512-531, 1967.

GOTTHEINER V. : Long-range strenuous sports training for cardiac reconditioning and rehabilitation. — Amer. J. Cardiol., 22 : 426-435, 1968.

GRAHAM T.P., ROSS J., COVELL J.W., SONNENBLICK E.H., CLANCY R.L. : Myocardial oxygen consumption in acute experimental cardiac depression. — Circulat. Res., 21 : 123-138, 1967.

GRIGGS D.M., TCHOKOEV V.V., CHEW C.C. : Transmural differences in ventricular tissue substrate levels due to coronary constriction. — Am. J. Physiol., 222 : 705-709, 1972.

GRIGGS D.M., TCHOKOEV V.V., DE CLUE J.W. : Non-uniform myocardial metabolism. — Circulation, 39, suppl. 3 : 96, 1969.

GRIMBY G. : Renal clearances during prolonged supine exercise at different loads. — *J. appl. Physiol.*, **20** : 1294-1298, 1965.

GRIMBY G., HÄGGENDAL E., SALTIN B. : Local Xenon[133] clearance from the quadriceps muscle during exercise in man. — *J. appl. Physiol.*, **22** : 305-310, 1967.

GRIMBY G., NILSSON N.J., SALTIN B. : Cardiac output during submaximal and maximal exercise in active middle-age athletes. — *J. appl. Physiol.*, **21** : 1150-1156, 1966.

GRIMBY G., SALTIN B. : Physiological effects of physical training. — *Scand. J. Rehab. Med.*, **3** : 6-14, 1971.

GUAZZI M., FIORENTINI C., POLESE A., MAGRINI F. : Continuous electrocardiographic recording in Prinzmetal's variant angina pectoris. A report of four cases. — *Brit Heart J.*, **32** : 611-616, 1970.

GUAZZI M., POLESE A., FIORENTINI C., MAGRINI F., BARTORELLI C. : Left ventricular performance and related hemodynamic changes in Prinzmetal's variant angina pectoris. — *Brit. Heart J.*, **33** : 84-94, 1971.

GUTMAN R.A., ALEXANDER E.R., LI Y.B., CHIANG B., WATTEN R.H., TING N., BRUCE R.A. : Delay of ST depression after maximal exercise by walking for 2 minutes. — *Circulation*, **42** : 229-233, 1970.

GUYTON A.C. : Regulation of cardiac output. — *New Engl. J. Med.*, **277** : 805-812, 1967.

HADDY F.J., SCOTT J.B. : Metabolically linked vasoactive chemicals in local regulation of blood flow. — *Physiol. Rev.*, **48** : 688-707, 1968.

HARRISON T.R., REEVES T.J. : Principles and problems of ischemic heart disease. Year Book Med. Publ., Chicago, 1968, 474 p.

HARTLEY L.H., GRIMBY G., KIBLOM A., NILSSON N.J., ÅSTRAND I., BJURE J., EKBLOM B., SALTIN B. : Physical training in sedentary middle-aged and older men. III. Cardiac output and gas exchange at submaximal and maximal exercise. — *Scand. J. clin. Lab. Invest.*, **24** : 335-344, 1969.

HARTLEY L.H., PERNOW B., HAGGENDAL J., LACOUR J., de LATTRE J., SALTIN B. : Central circulation during submaxmial work preceded by heavy exercise. — *J. appl. Physiol.*, **29** : 818-823, 1970.

HARTLEY L.H., SALTIN B. : Reduction of stroke volume and increase in heart rate after a previous heavier submaximal work load. — *Scand. J. clin. Lab. Invest.*, **22** : 217-223, 1968.

HELANDER E. : Economic aspects of the rehabilitation of patients with cardiovascular and cerebrovascular diseases. — *Acta Cardiol.*, suppl. 14 : 53-60, 1970.

HELFANT R.H., FORRESTER J.S., HAMPTON J.R., HAFT J.I., KEMP H.G., GORLIN R. : Coronary artery disease. Differential hemodynamic, metabolic and electrocardiographic effects in subjects with and whithout angina pectoris during atrial pacing. — *Circulation*, **42** : 601-610, 1970.

HELFANT R.H., HERMAN M.V., GORLIN R. : Abnormalities of left ventricular contraction induced by beta adrenergic blockade. — *Circulation*, **43** : 641-647, 1971a.

HELFANT R.H., de VILLA M.A., MEISTER S.G. : Effect of sustained isometric handgrip exercise on left ventricular performance. — *Circulation*, **44** : 982-993, 1971b.

HELLERSTEIN H.K. : Exercise therapy in coronary disease. — *Bull. N.Y. Acad. Med.*, **44** : 1028-1047, 1968.

HELLERSTEIN H.K., BURLANDO A., HIRSCH E.Z., PLOTKIN F.H., FEIL G.H., WINKLER O., MARIK S., MARGOLIS N. : Active physical reconditioning of coronary patients. — *Circulation*, **32**, suppl. 2, 110, 1965.

HELLERSTEIN H.K., HORNSTEN T.R. : Assessing and preparing the patient for return to a meaningfull and productive life. — *J. Rehab.*, **32** : 48-52, 1966.

HELLERSTEIN H.K., HORNSTEN T.R., GOLDBARG A., BURLANDO A.G., FRIEDMAN E.H., HIRSCH E.Z., MARIK S. : The influence of active conditioning upon subjects with coronary artery disease. — *Canad. med. Ass. J.*, **96** : 758-759, 1967.

HELLERSTEIN H.K., PROZAN G.B., DOAN A.E., HENDERSON J.A. : Two step exercise test as a test of cardiac function in chronic rheumatic heart disease and in arteriosclerotic heart disease with old myocardial infarction. — *Amer. J. Cardiol.*, **7** : 234-252, 1961.

HERMAN M.V., ELLIOT W.C., GORLIN R. : An electrocardiographic, anatomic, and metabolic study of zonal myocardial ischemia in coronary heart disease. — *Circulation*, **35** : 834-846, 1967.

HERMANSEN L., EKBLOM B., SALTIN B. : Cardiac output during submaximal and maximal treadmill and bicycle exercise. — *J. appl. Physiol.*, **29** : 82-86, 1970.

HERMANSEN L., SALTIN B. : Oxygen uptake during maximal treadmill and bicycle exercise. — *J. appl. Physiol.*, **26** : 31-37, 1969.

HILL A.V., LONG C.N.H., LUPTON H. : Muscular exercise, lactic acid and the supply and utilization of oxygen. — *Proc. roy. Soc. London*, **96** : 438-475, 1924.

HILLESTAD L., EIE H. : Coronary arteriography and angina pectoris. — *Acta med. scand.*, **188** : 425-430, 1970.

HINKLE L.E., CARVER S.T., STEVENS M. : The frequency of asymptomatic disturbances of cardiac rhythm and conduction in middle-aged men. — *Amer. J. Cardiol.*, **24** : 629-650, 1969.

HIRSCH E.Z. : The effects of digoxin on the electrocardiogram after strenuous exercise in normal men. — *Amer. Heart J.*, **70** : 196-203, 1965.

HOLLOSZY J.O. : Biochemical adaptations in muscle. Effects of exercise on mitochondrial oxygen uptake and respiratory enzyme activity in skeletal muscle. — *J. biol. Chem.*, **242** : 2278-2282, 1967.

HOLMGREN A., JONSSON B., SJOSTRAND T. : Circulatory data in normal subjects at rest and during exercise in recumbent position with special reference to the stroke volume at different work intensities. — *Acta physiol. Scand.*, **49** : 343-363, 1960.

HOLMGREN A., OVENFORS C.O. : Heart volume at rest and during muscular work in the supine and in the sitting position. — *Acta med. scand.*, **167** : 267-277, 1960.

HORNSTEN T.R., BRUCE R.A. : Computed ST forces of Frank and bipolar exercise electrocardiograms. -- *Amer. Heart J.*, **78** : 346-357, 1969.

HULTGREN H., CALCIANO A., PLATT F., ABRAMS H. : A clinical evaluation of coronary arteriography. — *Amer. J. Med.*, **42** : 228-247, 1967.

JAMES T.N. : Pathology of small coronary arteries. Review — *Amer. J. Cardiol.*, **20** : 679-691, 1967.

JAMES T.N. : Angina without coronary disease. — *Circulation*, **42** : 189-191, 1970.

JORGENSEN C.R., KITAMURA K., GOBEL F.L., TAYLOR H.T., WANG Y. : Long-term precision of the N₂O method for coronary flow during heavy upright exercise. — *J. appl. Physiol.*, **30** : 338-344, 1971.

JULIUS S., AMERY A., WHITLOCK L.S., CONWAY J. : Influence of age on the hemodynamic response to exercise. — *Circulation*, **36** : 222-230, 1967.

KAIJSER L. : Limiting factors for aerobic muscle performance. The influence of varying oxygen pressure and temperature. — *Acta physiol. Scand.*, **78**, suppl. 346, 1970, 96 p.

KAPLINSKI E., HOOD W.B., McCARTHY B., McCOMBS H.L., LOWN B. : Effects of physical training in dogs with coronary artery ligation. — *Circulation*, **37** : 556-565, 1968.

KASCH F.W., BOYER J.L. : Changes in maximum work capacity resulting from six months training in patients with ischemic heart disease. — *Med. Sci. Sports*, **1** : 156-159, 1969.

KASSEBAUM D.G., JUDKINS M.P., GRISWOLD H.E. : Stress electrocardiography in the evaluation of surgical revascularization of the heart. — *Circulation*, **40** : 297-313, 1969.

KASSEBAUM D.G., SUTHERLAND K.I., JUDKINS M.P. : A comparison of hypoxemia and exercise electrocardiography in coronary artery disease. Diagnostic precision of the methods correlated with coronary arteriography. — *Amer. Heart J.*, **75** : 758-776, 1968.

KASSER I.S., BRUCE R.A. : Comparative effects of aging and coronary heart disease on submaximal and maximal exercise. -- *Circulation*, **39** : 759-774, 1969.

KATZ L.N., FEINBERG H. : The relation of cardiac effort to myocardial oxygen consumption and coronary flow. — *Circulat. Res.*, **6** : 656-669, 1958.

KAWAI C., HULTGREN H.N. : The effect of digitalis upon the exercise electrocardiogram. — *Amer. Heart J.*, **68** : 409-420, 1964.

KEYS A. : Coronary heart disease in seven countries. — *Circulation*, **41**, suppl. 1 : 1-211, 1970a.

KEYS A. : Physical activity and the epidemiology of coronary heart disease. — *Med. Sport*, **4** : 250-266, 1970b.

KHAJA F., SANGHVI V., MARK A., PARKER J.O. : Effect of volume expansion on the angina treshold. — *Circulation*, **43** : 824-835, 1971.

KIBLOM A. : Physical training with submaximal intensities in women. I. Reaction to exercise and orthostasis. — *Scand. J. clin. Lab. Invest.*, **28** : 141-161, 1971.

KIBLOM A., ÅSTRAND I. : Physical training with submaximal intensities in women. II. Effect on cardiac output. — *Scand. J. clin. Lab. Invest.*, **28** : 163-175, 1971.

KIBLOM A., HARTLEY L.H., SALTIN B., BJURE I., BRIMBY G., ÅSTRAND I. : Physical training in sedentary middle-aged and older men. I. Medical evaluation. — *Scand. J. clin. Lab. Invest.*, **24** : 315-322, 1969.

KIESSLING K.H., PIEHL K., LUNDQUIST C.G. : Number and size of skeletal muscle mitochondria in trained sedentary men, p. 143-146 in LARSEN O.A., MALMBORG R.O. : Coronary heart disease and physical fitness, Munksgaard, Copenhagen, 1971, 277 p.

KINSELLA D., TROUP W., McGREGOR M. : Studies with a new coronary vasodilator drug : Persantin. -- *Amer. Heart J.*, **63** : 146-151, 1962.

KITAMURA K., JORGENSEN C.R., GOBEL F.L., TAYLOR H.L., WANG Y. : Hemodynamic correlates of coronary blood flow and myocardial oxygen consumption during upright exercise. — *Circulation*, **42** : 173, 1970.

KITZING J., KUTTA D., BLEICHERT A. : Temperaturregulation bei langdauernder schwerer körperlicher Arbeit. — *Pflüg. Arch.*, **301** : 241-253, 1968.

KIVOWITZ C., PARMLEY W.W., DONOSO R., MARCUS H., GANZ W., SWAN H.J.C. : Effects of isometric exercise on cardiac performance. The grip test. — *Circulation*, **44** : 994-1002, 1971.

KREMER R., TIMMERMANS G., BAUDREZ J., LAMBRECHT P. : Hémodynamique pulmonaire dans la pneumoconiose des houilleurs. — *Rev. Inst. Hyg. Mines*, **22** : 3-24, 1967.

KROEKER E.J., WOOD E.H. : Comparison of simultaneously recorded central and peripheral arterial pressure pulses during rest, exercise and tilted position in man. — *Circulat. Res.*, **3** : 623-632, 1955.

LAMMERANT J. : Circulation coronaire, in Proceedings of a session on the rehabilitation of coronary patients, W.H.O., Genève, 1972, in press.

LAU S.H., COHEN S.I., STEIN E., HAFT J.I., KINNEY M.J., YOUNG M.W., HELFANT R.H., DAMATO A.N. : Controlled heart rate by atrial pacing in angina pectoris. A determinant of electrocardiographic ST depression. — *Circulation*, **38** : 711-720, 1968.

LEON D.F., AMIDI M., LEONARD J.J. : Left heart work and temperature responses to cold exposure in man. — *Amer. J. Cardiol.*, **26** : 38-45, 1970.

LEPESCHKIN E., SURAWICZ B. : Characteristics of true-positive and false-positive results of electrocardiographic Master two-step exercise tests. — *New Engl. J. Med.*, **258** : 511-520, 1958.

LESTER F.M., SHEFFIELD L.T., REEVES T.J. : Electrocardiographic changes in clinically normal older men following near maximal and maximal exercise. — *Circulation*, **36** : 5-14, 1967.

LESTER M., SHEFFIELD L.T., TRAMMEL P., REEVES T.J. : The effect of age and athletic training on the maximal heart rate during muscular exercise. — *Amer. Heart J.*, **76** : 370-376, 1968.

LEUNISSEN R.L.A., PIATNEK-LEUNISSEN D.A., NAKAMURA Y., GRIGGS D.M. : Regional metabolism of the heart during reduced coronary flow. — *Circulation*, **24** : 155-156, 1966.

LEVINE J.H., NEILL W.A., WAGMAN R.J., KRASNOW N., GORLIN R. : The effect of exercise on mean left ventricular ejection rate in man. — *J. clin. Invest.*, **41** : 1050-1058, 1962.

LICHTLEN P. : La fonction du myocarde en cas de sclérose coronarienne. — *Triangle*, **9** : 282-292, 1970.

LICHTLEN P., ALBERT H., MOCCETTI T. : Left ventricular dynamics at rest and during exercise under different beta-blocking agents in patients with severe coronary artery disease. p. 205-221 in : KALTENBACH M., LICHTLEN P. : Coronary heart disease. Georg Thieme Verlag, Stuttgart, 1971, 271 p.

LIJESTRAND, STENSTRÖM : *Scand. Arch. Physiol.*, **39** : 167, 1920.

LIND A.R. : Cardiovascular responses to static exercise. — *Circulation*, **41** : 173-176, 1970.

LIND A.R., McNICOL G.W., DONALD K.W. : Circulatory adjustments to sustained (static) muscular activity, p. 38-63 in EVANG K., ANDERSEN K.L. : Physical activity in Health and Disease, Universiteitsforlaget, Oslo, 1966.

MacALPIN R.N., KATTUS A.A., WINFIELD M.E. : The effect of a beta-adrenergic-blocking agent (Nethalide) and nitroglycerin on exercise tolerance in angina pectoris. — *Circulation*, **31** : 869-875, 1965.

MAKOUS N., GITTLEMAN M.A., VALBUENA ATENCIO N.E. : The post two-step test electrocardiogram and hemodynamic determinants of myocardial oxygen consumption. — *Mal. Cardiovasc.*, **10** : 161-182, 1969.

MAKOUS N., HONG D.C., TAYLOR E.J. : Hemodynamics of the Master two-step test in hypertension and healed myocardial infarction. — *Circulation*, **30** : 77-85, 1964.

MALMBORG R.O. : A clinical and hemodynamic analysis of factors limiting the cardiac performance in patients with coronary heart disease. — *Acta med. scand.*, **177**, suppl. 426, 1964, 94 p.

MALMCRONA R., CRAMER G., VARNAUSKAS E. : Hemodynamic data during rest and exercise for patients who have or have nor been able to retain their occupation after myocardial infarction. — *Acta med. Scand.*, **174** : 557-572, 1963.

MANN G.V., GARRET H.L., FAHRI A., MURRAY H., BILLINGS F.T. : Exercise to prevent coronary heart disease. — *Amer. J. Med.*, **46** : 12-27, 1969.

MARSHALL R.J., SHEPHERD J.T. : Cardiac function in health and disease. W.B. Saunders Cy, Philadelphia, 1968, 409 p.

MASON D.T., BRAUNWALD E. : The effects of nitroglycerin and amyl nitrite on arteriolar and venous tone in the human forearm. — *Circulation*, **32** : 755-766, 1965.

MASON D.T., SPANN J.F., ZELIS R., AMSTERDAM E.A. : Physiological approach to the treatment of angina pectoris. — *N. Engl. J. Med.*, **281** : 1225-1228, 1969.

MASON R.E., LIKAR I. : A new system of multiple lead exercise electrocardiography. — *Amer. Heart J.*, **71** : 196-205, 1966.

MASON R.E., LIKAR I., BIERN R.O., ROSS R.S. : Multiple-lead exercise electrocardiography. Experience in 107 normal subjects and 67 patients with angina pectoris, and comparison with coronary cinearteriography in 84 patients. — *Circulation*, **36** : 517-525, 1967.

MASTER A.M. : The Master two-step test. — *Amer. Heart J.*, **75** : 809-837, 1968.

MASTER A.M. : ST elevation. — *Amer. Heart J.*, **80** : 434, 1970.

MASTER A.M., FRIEDMAN R., DACK S. : The electrocardiogram after standard exercise as a functional test of the heart. — *Amer. Heart J.*, **24** : 777-793, 1942.

MASTER A.M., ROSENFELD I. : Criteria for the clinical application of the « two-step » exercise test. Obviation of false-negative and false-positive responses. — *J. Amer. med. Ass.*, 178 : 283-289, 1961.

MATTINGLY T.W. : The potexercise electrocardiogram. Its value in the diagnosis and prognosis of coronary arterial disease. — *Amer. J. Cardiol.*, **9** : 395-409, 1962.

McCONAHAY D.R., McCALLISTER B.D., SMITH R.E. : Postexercise electrocardiography : correlations with coronary arteriography and left ventricular hemodynamics. — *Amer. J. Cardiol.*, **28** : 1-9, 1971.

McDONOUGH J.R., KUSUMI F., BRUCE R.A. : Variations in maximal oxygen intake with physical activity in middle-aged men. — *Circulation*, **41** : 743-751, 1970.

McHENRY P.L., FISCH C., JORDAN J.W., CORYA B.R. : Cardiac arrhythmias observed during maximal treadmill exercise testing in clinically normal men. — *Am. J. Cardiol.*, **29** : 331-336, 1972.

McHENRY P.L., STOWE D.E., LANCASTER M.C. : Computer quantitation of the ST-segment response during maximal treadmill exercise. Clinical correlation. — *Circulation*, **38** : 691-701, 1968.

MESSER J.V., LEVINE H.J., WAGMAN R.J., GORLIN R. : Effect of exercise on cardiac performance in human subjects with coronary artery disease. — *Circulation*, 28 : 404-414, 1963.

MESSER J.V., WAGMAN R.J., LEVINE H.J., NEILL W.A., KRASNOW N., GORLIN R. : Patterns of human myocardial oxygen extraction during rest and exercise. — *J. clin. Invest.*, 41 : 725-742, 1962.

MESSIN R., DENOLIN H., DEGRE S. : Etude d'un test simple d'aptitude à l'effort : la CT 170. — *Arch. Mal. Cœur*, 3, 305-316, 1965.

MICHAEL E.D., HUTTON K.E., HORVATH S.M. : Cardiocirculatory responses during prolonged exercise. — *J. appl. Physiol.*, 16 : 997-1000, 1961.

MITCHELL J.H., SPROULE B.J., CHAPMAN C.B. : The physiological meaning of the maximal oxygen intake test. — *J. clin. Invest.*, 37 : 538-547, 1958.

MJÖS O.D. : Effect of free fatty acids on myocardial function and oxygen consumption in intact dogs.. — *J. clin. Invest.*, 50 : 1386-1389, 1971.

MJÖS O.D., KJEKSHUS J. : Increased local metabolic rate by free fatty acids in the intact dog heart. — *Scand. J. clin. Lab. Invest.*, 28 : 389-393, 1971.

MONROE R.G. : Myocardial oxygen consumption during ventricular contraction and relaxation. — *Circulat. Res.*, 14 : 294-300, 1964.

MORGAN T.E., SHORT F.A., COBB L.A. : Effect of long-term exercise on skeletal muscle lipid composition. — *Amer. J. Physiol.*, 216 : 82-86, 1969.

MOSS A.J. : Intramyocardial oxygen tension. — *Cardiovasc. Res.*, 2 : 314-318, 1968.

MOST A.S., KEMP H.G., GORLIN R. : Postexercise electrocardiography in patients with arteriographically documented coronary artery disease. — *Ann. int. Med.*, 71 : 1043-1049, 1969.

MULHAUSEN R.O. : The affinity of hemoglobin for oxygen. — *Circulation*, 42 : 195-198, 1970.

MÜLLER O., RORVIK K. : Hemodynamic consequences of coronary heart disease. — *Brit. Heart J.*, 20 : 302-310, 1958.

MULLINS C.B., LESHIN S.J., MIERZWIAK D.S., MATTHEWS O.A., BLOMQVIST C.G. : Isometric exercise (handgrip) as a stress test for evaluation of left ventricular function. — *Circulation*, 42, suppl. 3 : 122, 1970.

NAJMI F., GRIGGS D.M. Jr., KASPARIAN H., NOVACK P. : Effects of nitroglycerin on hemodynamics during rest and exercise in patients with coronary insufficiency. — *Circulation*, 35 : 46-54, 1967.

NASSER M.G. : The coronary system, p. 261-292 in RUSHMER R.F. : Cardiovascular dynamics, W.B. Saunders Cy, Philadelphia, 1970, 559 p.

NAUGHTON J., NAGLE F. : Peak oxygen intake during physical fitness program for middle-aged men. — *J. Amer. med. Ass.*, 191 : 103-105, 1965.

NAUGHTON J., SHANBOUR K., ARMSTRONG R. McCOY J., LATEGOLA M.T. : Cardiovascular respons' to exercise following myocardial infarction. — *Arch. int Med.*, 117 : 541-545, 1966.

NEIL W.A. : Myocardial hypoxia and anaerobic metabol'sm in coronary heart disease. — *Amer. J. Cardiol.*, 22 : 507-515, 1968.

NORMAND J., DELAYE J., LOUISOT P., CAHEN P., AMIEL M., SILIE M., FROMENT R. : L'angine de poitrine à coronarographie normale. Critères de diagnostic et hypothèses pathogéniques. Mise en évidence d'anomalies enzymatiques myocardiques. — *Arch. Mal. Cœur.*, 64 : 1689-1710, 1971.

O'BRIEN K.P., HIGGS L.M., GLANCY D.L., EPSTEI S.E. : Hemodynamic accompaniments of angina : a com parison during angina induced by exercise and by atrial pacing. — *Circulation*, 39 : 735-743, 1969.

PARKER J.O., CASE R.B., KHAJA F., LEDWICH J.R., ARMSTRONG P.W. : The influence of changes in blood volume on angina pectoris. A study of the effect of phlebotomy. — *Circulation*, 41 : 593-604, 1970a.

PARKER J.O., CHIONG M.A., WEST R.O., CASE R.B. : Sequential alterations in myocardial lactate metabolism, ST segments, and left ventricular function during angina induced by atrial pacing. — *Circulation*, 40 : 113-131, 1969b.

PARKER J.O., CHIONG M.A., WEST R.O., CASE R.B. : The effect of ischemia and alterations in heart rate on myocardial potassium balance in man. — *Circulation*, 42 : 205-217, 1970b.

PARKER J.O., Di GIORGI S., WEST R.O. : Hemodynamic study of acute coronary insufficiency precipitated by exercise : with observations on the effects of nitroglycerin. — *Amer. J. Cardiol.*, 17 : 470-483, 1966.

PARKER J.O., LEDWICH J.R., WEST R.O., CASE R.B. : Reversible cardiac failure during angina pectoris. Hemodynamic effects of atrial pacing in coronary artery disease. — *Circulation*, 39 : 745-757, 1969a.

PARKER J.O., WEST R.O., Di GIORGI S. : The hemodynamic response to exercise in patients with healed myocardial infarction without angina. With observations on the effects of nitroglycerin. — *Circulation*, 36 : 734-751, 1967.

PARKER J.O., WEST R.O., Di GIORGI S. : The effect of nitroglycerin on coronary blood flow and the hemodynamic response to exercise in coronary artery disease. — *Amer. J. Cardiol.*, 27 : 59-65, 1971.

PIETTE F., DETRY J.M., BRASSEUR L.A. : Physiopathologie de l'angor d'effort. Implications thérapeutiques. — *Louvain Méd.*, 89 : 149-163, 1970.

PIRNAY F., DEROANNE R., PETIT J.M. : Maximal oxygen consumption in a hot environment. — *J. appl. Physiol.*, 218 : 642-645, 1970a.

PIRNAY F., DEROANNE R., PETIT J.M., BOTTIN R., DUJARDIN J. : Signification de la consommation d'oxygène correspondant à la fréquence cardiaque de 170/min. — *Int. Z. angew. Physiol.*, 29 : 1-10, 1970b.

PIRNAY F., LAMY M., DUJARDIN J., DEROANNE R., PETIT J.M. : Analysis of femoral venous blood during maximum muscular exercise. — *J. appl. Physiol.*, in press, 1972.

PIRNAY F., PETIT J.M., BOTTIN R., DEROANNE R., JUCHMES J., BELGE J. : Comparaison de deux méthodes de mesure de la consommation maximum d'oxygène. — *Int. Z. angew. Physiol.*, 23 : 203-211, 1966.

PRINZMETAL M., EKMECKI A., KENNAMER R., KWOCZYNSKI J.K., SHUBIN H., TOYOSHIMA H. : Variant from of angina pectoris. Perviously undelineated syndrome. — *J. Amer. med. Ass.*, 174 : 1794-1800, 1960.

PROFANT G.R., EARLY R.G., NILSON K.L., KUSUMI F., BRUCE R.A. : Aerobic capacity, circulatory and electrocardiographic responses to maximal exercise in healthy middle-aged women. Personnal Communication, 1971.

PROUDFIT W.L., SHIREY E.K., SONES F.M. : Selective cine-coronary arteriography. Correlation with clinical findings in 1000 patients. — *Circulation*, 33 : 901-910, 1966.

PUNSAR S., PYÖRÄLÄ K., SILTANEN P. : Classification of electrocardiographic ST segment changes in epidemiological studies of coronary heart disease. Preliminary evaluation of a new modified classification, with particular reference to the prognostic significance of different types of ST segment changes. — *Ann. med. int. Fenn.*, 57 : 53-63, 1968.

PYFER H.R., DOAN B.L. : Cardiac arrest during exercise training. Report of a successfully treated case attributed to preparedness. — *J. Amer. med. Ass.*, 210 : 101-102, 1969.

PYÖRÄLÄ K., KÄRÄVÄ R., PUNSAR S., OJA P., TERÄSLINNA P., PARTANEN T., JÄÄSKELÄINEN M., PEKKARINEN M-L., KOSKELA A. : A controlled study of the effects of 18 month's physical training in sedentary middle-aged men with high indexes of risk relative to coronary heart disease, p. 261-265 in LARSEN O.A., MALMBORG R.O. : Coronary heart disease and physical fitness, Munksgaard, Copenhagen, 1971, 277 p.

PYÖRÄLÄ M.J., KARVONEN M.J., TASKINEN P., TAKKUNEN J., KYRÖNSEPPÄ H., PELTOKALLIO P. : Cardiovascular studies on former endurance athletes. — *Amer. J. Cardiol.*, 20 : 191-205, 1967.

RECHNITZER P.A., PICKARD H.A., PAIVIO A.U., YUHASZ M.S., CUNNINGHAM D. : Longterm follow-up study of survival and recurrence rates following myocardial infarction in exercising and control subjects. — *Circulation*, 45 : 853-857, 1972.

REDWOOD D.R., ROSING D.R., GOLSTEIN R.E., BEISER G.D., EPSTEIN S.E. : Importance of the design of an exercise protocol in the evaluation of patients with angina pectoris. — *Circulation*, 43 : 618-628, 1971.

REEVES J.T., GROVER R.F., BLOUNT S.G., FILLEY G.F. : Cardiac output response to standing and treadmill walking. — *J. appl. Physiol.*, 16 : 283-288, 1961b.

REEVES J.T., GROVER R.F., FILLEY G.F., BLOUNT S.G. : Circulatory changes in man during mild supine exercise. — *J. appl. Physiol.*, 16 : 279-282, 1961a.

REINDELL H., KÖNIG K., ROSKAMM H. : Funktionsdiagnostik des gesunden und kranken Herzens. Thieme Verlag, Stuttgart, 1967, 294 p.

ROBB G.P., MARKS H.H. : Latent coronary artery disease. Determination of its presence and severity by the exercise electrocardiogram. — *Amer. J. Cardiol.*, 13 : 603-618, 1964.

ROBINSON B.F. : Relation of heart rate and systolic blood pressure to the onset of the pain in angina pectoris. — *Circulation*, 35 : 1073-1083, 1967.

ROBINSON B.F. : Mode af action of nitroglycerin in angina pectoris. Correlation between haemodynamic effects during exercise and prevention of pain. — *Brit. Heart J.*, 30 : 295-302, 1968.

ROBINSON S. : Experimental studies of physical fitness in relation to age. — *Arbeitsphysiologie*, 10 : 251-323, 1938.

ROBINSON S. : Training, acclimatization and heat tolerance. — *Canad. med. Ass. J.*, 96 : 795-799, 1967.

ROCHMIS P., BLACKBURN H. : Exercise test : a survey of procedures, safety and litigation experience in approximately 170 000 tests. — *J. Amer. med. Ass.*, 1061-1066, 1971.

ROITMAN D., JONES W.B., SHEFFIELD L.T. : Comparison of submaximal exercise ECG test with coronary cineangiogram. — *Ann. int. Med.*, 72 : 641-647, 1970.

ROSELLE H.A., CRAMPTON R.S., CASE R.B. : Alternans of the depressed ST segment during coronary insufficiency. Its relation to mechanical events. — *Amer. J. Cardiol.*, 18 : 200-207, 1966.

ROSKAMM H. : Optimum patterns of exercise for healthy adults. — *Canad. med. Ass. J.*, 96 : 895-900, 1967.

ROSLAND G.A. : Hemodynamic observations during spontaneous angina pectoris. — *Brit. Heart J.*, 31 : 523-525, 1969.

ROUGHGARDEN J.W. : Circulatory changes associated with spontaneous angina pectoris. — *Amer. J. Med.*, 41 : 947-961, 1966.

ROUSSEAU M., BRASSEUR L.A. : Critères d'arrêt des épreuves d'effort. — *Acta Cardiol.*, 27 : 392-406, 1972.

ROUSSEAU M., BRASSEUR L.A., DETRY J-M. R. : Hemodynamic and electrocardiographic effects of practolol during exercise in coronary heart disease. In press : *Cardiovasc. Res.*, 1972a.

ROUSSEAU M., VANDENBROUCKE G., DETRY J.M.R., BRASSEUR L.A. : Hemodynamic effects of physical training in coronary heart disease. In preparation, 1972b.

ROWE G.G., CHELIUS C.J., AFONSO S., GURTNER H.P., CRUMPTON C.W. : Systemic and coronary hemodynamic effects of erythrol tetranitrate. — *J. clin. Invest.*, 40 : 1217-1222, 1961.

ROWELL L.B. : Factors affecting the prediction of the maximal oxygen intake from measurements made during submaximal work with observations related to factors which may limit maximal oxygen intake. Ph. D. Thesis, University of Minnesota, Minneapolis, 1962, 275 p.

ROWELL L.B. : Circulation. — *Med. Sci. Sports*, 1 : 15-22, 1969.

ROWELL L.B. : Distribution of cardiac output during exercise and the effect of training, p. 57-61 in LARSEN O.A., MALMBORG R.O. : Coronary heart disease and physical fitness, Munksgaard, Copenhagen, 1971, 277 p.

ROWELL L.B., BLACKMON J.R., BRUCE R.A. : Indocyanine green clearance and estimated hepatic blood flow during mild to maximal exercise in upright man. — *J. clin. Invest.*, 43 : 1677-1690, 1964a.

ROWELL L.B., BRENGELMANN G.L., BLACKMON J.R., BRUCE R.A., MURRAY J.A. : Disparities between aortic and peripheral pulse pressures induced by upright exercise and vasomotor changes in man. — *Circulation*, 37 : 954-964, 1968.

ROWELL L.B., BRENGELMANN G.L., DETRY J.M., R., WYSS C. : Venomotor responses to rapid changes in skin temperature in exercising man. — *J. appl. Physiol.*, 30 : 64-71, 1971a.

ROWELL L.B., BRENGELMANN G.L., DETRY J-M. R., WYSS C. : Venomotor responses to local and remote thermal stimuli to skin in exercising man. — *J. appl. Physiol.*, 30 : 72-77, 1971b.

ROWELL L.B., KRANING K.K., KENNEDY J.W., EVANS T.O. : Central circulatory responses to work in dry heat before and after acclimatization. — *J. appl. Physiol.*, 22 : 509-518, 1967.

ROWELL L.B., MARX H.J., BRUCE R.A., CONN R.D., KUSUMI F. : Reductions in cardiac output, central blood volume, and stroke volume with thermal stress in normal men during exercise. — *J. clin. Invest.*, 45 : 1801-1816, 1966.

ROWELL L.B., MURRAY J.A., BRENGELMANN G.L., KRANING K.K. : Human cardiovascular adjustments to rapid changes in skin temperature during exercise. — *Circulat. Res.*, 24 : 711-724, 1969.

ROWELL L.B., TAYLOR H.L., SIMONSON E., CARLSON W.S. : The physiologic fallacy of adjusting for body weight in performance of the Master two-step test. — *Amer. Heart J.*, 70 : 461-465, 1965.

ROWELL L.B., TAYLOR H.L., WANG Y. : Limitations to prediction of maximal oxygen intake. — *J. appl. Physiol.*, 19 : 919-927, 1964c.

ROWELL L.B., TAYLOR H.L., WANG Y., CARLSON W.S. : Saturation of arterial blood with oxygen during maximal exercise. — *J. appl. Physiol.*, 19 : 284-286, 1964b.

RUBIO R., BERNE R.M. : Release of adenosine by the normal myocardium in dogs and its relationship to the regulation of coronary resistance. — *Circulat. Res.*, 25 : 407-415, 1969.

RUMBALL A., ACHESON E.D. : Latent coronary heart disease detected by electrocardiogram before and after exercise. — *Brit. Med. J.*, 1 : 423-428, 1963.

RUSSEK H.I. : Master two-step test in coronary artery disease. — *J. Amer. med. Ass.*, 165 : 1772-1775, 1957.

RUSSEK H.I. : Propranolol and isorbide dinitrate synergism in angina pectoris. — *Amer. J. Cardiol.*, 21 : 44-54, 1968.

SALTIN B. : Circulatory response to submaximal and maximal exercise after thermal dehydratation. — *J. appl. Physiol.*, 19 : 1125-1132, 1964a.

SALTIN B. : Aerobic work capacity and circulation at exercise in man. With special reference to the effect of prolonged exercise and/or heat exposure. — *Acta physiol. Scand.*, 62, suppl. 230, 1964b, 52 p.

SALTIN B. : Physiological effects of physical conditioning. — *Med. Sci. Sports*, 1 : 50-56, 1969.

SALTIN B., ÅSTRAND P.O. : Maximal oxygen uptake in athletes. — *J. appl. Physiol.*, 23 : 353-358, 1967.

SALTIN B., BLOMQVIST G.M., MITCHELL J.H., JOHNSON R.L., WILDENTHAL K., CHAPMAN C.B. : Response to exercise after bedrest and after training. — *Circulation*, 38, suppl. 7, 1968, 78 p.

SALTIN B., GRIMBY G. : Physiological analysis of middle aged and old former athletes : comparison with still active athletes of the same ages. — *Circulation*, 38 : 1104-1115, 1968.

SALTIN B., HARTLEY L.H., KIBLOM A., ÅSTRAND I. : Physical training in sedentary middle-aged and older men. II. Oxygen uptake, heart rate, and blood lactate concentration at submaximal and maximal exercise. — *Scand. J. clin. Lab. Invest.*, 24 : 323-334, 1969.

SALTIN B., STENBERG J. : Circulatory response to prolonged severe exercise. — *J. appl. Physiol.*, 19 : 833-838, 1964.

SALZMAN S.H., HELLERSTEIN H.K., RADKE J.D., MAISTELMAN H.W., RICKLIN R. : Quantitative effects of physical conditioning on the exercise electrocardiogram of middle-aged subjects with arteriosclerotic heart disease, p. 388-410 in : Measurement in exercise electrocardiography, C.C. Thomas, Springfield, 1969, 488 p.

SAMPSON J.J., CHEITLIN M.D. : Pathophysiology and differential diagnosis of cardiac pain. — *Prog. Cardiovasc. Dis.*, 13 : 507-531, 1971.

SARNOFF S.J., BRAUNWALD E., WELCH G.H., CASE R.B., STAINSBY W.N., MACRUZ R. : Hemodynamic determinants of oxygen consumption of the heart with special reference to the tension-time-index. — *Amer. J. Physiol.*, 192 : 148-156, 1958.

SCANDINAVIAN COMMITTEE on ECG classification : The « Minnesota code » for ECG classification. Adaptation to CR leads and modification of the code for ECGs recorded during and after exercise. — *Acta med. scand.*, 181, suppl. 481 : 1967, 26 p.

SCHEUER J. : Myocardial metabolism in cardiac hypoxia. — *Amer. J. Cardiol.*, 19 : 385-392, 1967.

SHAPPELL S.D., MURRAY J.A., NASSER M.G., WILLS R.E., TORRANCE J.D., LENFANT C.J.M. : Acute change in hemoglobin affinity for oxygen during angina pectoris. — *N. England J. Med.,* 282 : 1219-1224, 1970.

SHEFFIELD L.T., HOLT J.H., LESTER F.M., CONROY D.V., REEVES T.J. : On-line analysis of the exercise electrocardiogram. — *Circulation,* 40 : 935-944, 1969.

SHEFFIELD L.T., HOLT J.H., REEVES T.J. : Exercise graded by heart rate in electrocardiographic testing for angina pectoris. — *Circulation,* 32 : 622-629, 1965.

SHELDON W.C. : On the significance of coronary collaterals. — *Amer. J. Cardiol.,* 24 : 303-304, 1969.

SHEPHARD R.J., ALLEN C., BENADE A.J.S., DAVIES C.T.M., di PRAMPERO P.E., HEDMAN R., MERRIMAN J.E., MYHRE K., SIMMONS R. : The maximum oxygen intake. An international reference standard of cardiorespiratory fitness. — *Bull. Wld. Hlth. Org.,* 38 : 757-764, 1968.

SHEPHERD J.T. : Behavior of resistance and capacity vessels in human limbs during exercise. — *Circulat. Res.,* 20 : 70-81, 1967.

SHORT F.A., ROSS R., COBB L.A., MORGAN T.E. : The induction of human muscle mitochondrial proliferation and increased glycogen and triglyceride synthesis by long-term exercise. — *J. clin. Invest.,* 49 : 88a-89a, 1970.

SIEGEL W., BLOMQVIST G., MITCHELL J.H. : Effects of a quantitated physical training program on middle-age sedentary men. — *Circulation,* 41 : 19-29, 1970.

SIMONSON E. : Electrocardiographic stress tolerance tests. — *Prog. Cardiovasc. Dis.,* 13 : 269-292, 1970.

SJÖSTRAND T. : Changes in the respiratory organs of workmen at an ore smelting works. — *Acta med. scand.,* suppl. 196 : 687-691, 1947.

SKINNER N.S., POWELL W.J. : Regulation of skeletal muscle blood flow during exercise. Action of oxygen and potassium. — *Circulat. Res.,* 20, suppl. 1 : 59-67, 1967.

SOLVAY H., DENOLIN H. : L'électrocardiogramme d'effort. Technique et interprétation. Hôpital Universitaire Saint-Pierre, Bruxelles, 1967, 115 p.

SONNENBLICK E.H., ROSS J., BRAUNWALD E. : Oxygen consumption of the heart. Newer concepts of its multifactorial determination. — *Amer. J. Cardiol.,* 22 : 328-336, 1968.

SONNENBLICK E.H., ROSS J., COVELL J.W., KAISER G.A., BRAUNWALD E. : Velocity of contraction as a determinant of myocardial oxygen consumption. — *Amer. J. Physiol.,* 209 : 919-927, 1965.

SOWTON E., BALCON R., CROSS D., FRICK M.H. : Measurement of the angina treshold using atrial pacing. A new technique for the study of angina pectoris. — *Cardiovasc. Res.,* 1 : 301-307, 1967.

SOWTON E., BURKART F. : Hemodynamic changes during continuous exercise. — *Brit. Heart J.,* 29 : 770-774, 1967.

SOWTON E., SMITHEN C., LEAVER D., BARR I. : Effects of practolol on exercise tolerance in patients with angina pectoris. — *Amer. J. Med.,* 51 : 63-70, 1971.

STENBERG J., ÅSTRAND P.O., EKBLOM B., ROYCE J., SALTIN B. : Hemodynamic response to work with different muscle groups sitting and supine. — *J. appl. Physiol.,* 22 : 61-70, 1967.

STRANDELL T. : Circulatory studies of healthy old men. — *Acta med. scand.,* 175, suppl. 414, 1964, 44 p.

TABAKIN B.S., HANSON J.S., LEVY A.M. : Effects of physical training on the cardiovascular and respiratory response to graded upright exercise in distance runners. — *Brit. Heart J.,* 27 : 205-210, 1965.

TAYLOR H.L., BUSKIRK E., HENSCHEL A. : Maximal oxygen intake as an objective measure of cardio-respiratory performance. — *J. appl. Physiol.,* 8 : 73-80, 1955.

TAYLOR H.L., HASKELL W., FOX S.M., BLACKBURN H. : Exercise tests : a summary of procedures and concepts of stress testing for cardiovascular diagnosis and functional evaluation, p. 259-296 in BLACKBURN H. : Measurements in exercise electrocardiography, C.C. Thomas, Springfield, 1969, 488 p.

THOMAS C.B. : The cardiovascular response of normal young adults to exercise as determined by the double Master two-step test. Bull. Johns Hopk. Hosp., 89 : 181-217, 1951.

TRAP-JENSEN J., CLAUSEN J.P. : Effect of training on the relation of heart rate and blood pressure to the onset of pain in effort angina pectoris, p. 111-114 in LARSEN O.A., MALMBORG R.O. : Coronary heart disease and physical fitness, Munksgaard, Copenhagen, 1971, 277 p.

TUNA N., AMPLATZ K. : The significance of coronary collateral circulation. Coronary arteriographic and electrovectocardiographic correlations. — *Amer. J. Cardiol.,* 26 : 663, 1970.

UNTERMAN D., DE GRAFF A.C. : The effect of exercise on the electrocardiogram (Master « two-step » test) in the diagnosis of coronary insufficiency. — *Amer. J. med. Sci.,* 215 : 671-685, 1948.

VANDENBROUCKE G. : Programme de réadaptation physique de l'infarctus myocardique. — *Rev. Réadapt.,* 13 : 86-95, 1971.

VARNAUSKAS E., BERGMAN H., HOUK P., BJÖRNTORP P. : Haemodynamic effects of physical training in coronary patients. — *Lancet,* 2 : 8-12, 1966.

VARNAUSKAS E., BJÖRNTORP P., FAHLEN M., PREROVSKY I., STENBERG J. : Effects of physical training on exercise blood flow and enzymatic activity in skeletal muscle. — *Cardiovasc. Res.,* 4 : 418-422, 1970.

WADE O.L., BISHOP J.M. : Cardiac output and regional blood flow. Blackwell, Oxford, 1962, 268 p.

WALHUND H.G. : Determination of the physiological working capacity. — *Acta med. scand.,* **132,** suppl. 215, 1948, 36 p.

WANG Y., MARSHALL R.J., SHEPHERD J.T. : The effect of changes in posture and graded exercise on stroke volume in man. — *J. clin. Invest.,* **39** : 1051-1061, 1960.

WAXLER E.B., KIMBIRIS B., DREIFUS L.S. : The fate of women with normal coronary arteriograms and chest pain resembling angina pectoris. — *Amer. J. Cardiol.,* **28** : 25-32, 1971.

WIENER L., DWYER E.M. Jr., COX J.W. : Hemodynamic effects of nitroglycerin, propranolol, and their combination in coronary heart disease. —*Circulation,* **39** : 623-632, 1969.

WILKINS R.W., HAYNES F.W., WEISS S. : The role of the venous system in circulatory collapse induced by sodium nitrite. — *J. clin. Invest.,* **16** : 85-91, 1937.

WILLIAMS C.G., BREDELL G.A.G., WYNDHAM C.H., STRYDOM N.B., MORRISON J.F., PETER J., FLEMING P.W., WARD J.S. : Circulatory and metabolic reactions to work in heat. — *J. appl. Physiol.,* **17** : 625-638, 1962.

WILLIAMS J.F., GLICK G., BRAUNWALD E. : Studies on cardiac dimensions in intact unanesthetized man. V. Effects of nitroglycerin. — *Circulation,* **32** : 767-771, 1965.

WINBURY M.M., WEISS H.R., HOWE B.B. : Effects of beta-adrenoceptor blockade and nitroglycerin on myocardial oxygenation. — *Europ. J. Pharmacol.,* **16** : 271-277, 1971.

WONG H.O., KASSER I.S., BRUCE R.A. : Impaired maximal exercise performance with hypertensive cardiovascular disesae. — *Circulation,* **39** : 633-638, 1969.

WOOD P., McGREGOR M., MAGIDSON O., WHITTAKER W. : The effort test in angina pectoris. — *Brit. Heart J.,* **12** : 363-371, 1950.

GPSR Compliance

*The European Union's (EU) General Product Safety Regulation (GPSR)
is a set of rules that requires consumer products to be safe and our
obligations to ensure this.*

*If you have any concerns about our products, you can contact us on
ProductSafety@springernature.com*

In case Publisher is established outside the EU, the EU authorized
representative is:

Springer Nature Customer Service Center GmbH
Europaplatz 3
69115 Heidelberg, Germany

Batch number: 09635766

Printed by Printforce, the Netherlands